LISTEN: HEALTHY PERSON TALKING

LISTEN: HEALTHY PERSON TALKING

Frederick Mickel Huck

authorHOUSE®

AuthorHouse™
1663 Liberty Drive
Bloomington, IN 47403
www.authorhouse.com
Phone: 1 (800) 839-8640

Published by AuthorHouse 08/19/2015

Library of Congress Control Number: 2015913660

ISBN: 978-1-5049-3291-2 (sc)
ISBN: 978-1-5049-3292-9 (e)

Print information available on the last page.

Any people depicted in stock imagery provided by Thinkstock are models, and such images are being used for illustrative purposes only. Certain stock imagery © Thinkstock.

This book is printed on acid-free paper.

Because of the dynamic nature of the Internet, any web addresses or links contained in this book may have changed since publication and may no longer be valid. The views expressed in this work are solely those of the author and do not necessarily reflect the views of the publisher, and the publisher hereby disclaims any responsibility for them.

CONTENTS

This book is dedicated to:

ROBERT E MENZIE

INEZ A MENZIE

DONALD W HUCK

AURA V HUCK

DR EDE KOENIG

Special thanks to:

Sandra V Mooney

Matthew F Mooney

John Dunlap

Angie Ingersoll

SOME BENEFITS OF BEING HEALTHY

It goes without saying that good health is the most important factor of life even a lot more important than money; money cannot buy good health. Good health can only be accomplished by knowledge and the commitment to act properly. Here are just a few reasons of the benefits of being healthy:

(1)   Enjoying the best of foods.

(2)   Having extra money to spend and save as your cost of living will be decreased.

(3)   Having extra discretion time to do other meaningful things.

(4)   Eliminating practically all illness and sickness.

(5)   The ability to make better mental decisions and problem solving activities will be increased.

(6)   A higher quality of life will be realized.

(7)   The need of expensive drugs will be practically eliminated.

(8)   Expensive and time consuming visits to the doctors and hospitals will be so rare as to be almost non existent.

(9)   Muscle strength and physical endurance will be increased.

(10)   A healthy body will increase ones appetite for meals and a variety of meals; and decrease the temptation to snack between meals.

(11)   And the excitement of being healthy will make you want to share your success with others.

OPINIONS ABOUT HEALTH FROM THE UNHEALTHY

During the last year of researching facts on what makes people healthy I have also researched views from unhealthy people in the hope of learning from the mistakes that brought on their illnesses. The following statements have been voiced by doctors, nurses, specialists, patients, and friends of patients, who have contributed to the horrible health of many people in the western world.

1. It is common that my body is malfunctioning because of my age.

2. A healthy person should receive regular check ups that include flu shots, and vaccines to maintain good health and prevent disease.

3. It is wise and healthy to take all drugs that are prescribed by a medical doctor, because they have advanced health degrees and know what is best for my health.

4. Health insurance is important for good health in case I get sick and will help me to regain good health in case of sickness.

5. People living in the United States have the best health care in the world.

6. Being overweight is beneficial because it will help a person survive an illness that may kill a slender person.

7. The Federal Drug Administration (FDA) will protect the population of the USA, from bad drugs that may be produced by the drug companies.

8. It is natural and normal to suffer from the flu or common colds once in a while, it is just part of normal life.

9. A person with cancer can function normally if under a doctor's care and after a time the cancer will go into remission, but the only hope that a person with cancer has is to find a good doctor.

10. Drug companies are respectful businesses because they give away drugs to the poor.

11. People in other countries die needlessly from diseases because those countries lack modern medical services.

12. Herbs, minerals, and natural methods of health care are not to be trusted because the FDA has not given their stamp of approval for these unconventional methods.

13. There is a shortage of doctors and nurses in the U.S.

14. Big drug companies are constantly looking for new cures for all diseases.

15. Cancer is not caused by X-rays.

16. The lack of drugs have historically caused epidemics to occur.

17. It is not harmful to eat junk food or drink alcohol if done in moderation.

18. There is good and bad cholesterol in everyone's bodies.

19. Very few people have worms or parasites in their bodies.

20. Medical foundations, like the Heart Foundation, Diabetes Foundation, and the Cancer Foundation are lacking funds to help cure the diseases.

21. No proof has ever been established to prove that government approved pesticides or herbicides are harmful to the human body.

22. The genes a person inherits from their parents is the biggest determination of the health of a person.

23. Getting enough exercise guarantees good health.

24. A person's blood type determines if he can consume meat and be healthy.

25. Air pollution is the reason most people are unhealthy.

26. If a person is hospitalized he will be healthier if he stays longer before he is released.

27. New drugs need to be developed to ensure healthier people.

28. A person with cancer can still be a healthy person.

29. Smoking cigarettes may not be healthy, but I will be happy when I die.

GUIDE 14 DAYS

The e purpose of this fourteen day meal plan is to illustrate that starvation does not exist when following the plan. Instead of listing the fruit on a daily log every day, I just list here approximately, what was eaten.

For the last three years, I have reversed my two meals. The larger was consumed first and the second is mostly raw. Prior to eating breakfast, generally a half an hour after I wake, I drink a quart of warm water with two teaspoons of lemon juice, one tablespoon of inland sea water and one tablespoon of silver mineral water. I consume approximately five pounds of fruit daily, and the fruit varies according to the seasons of the year.

The fourteen days are very similar (fruit meal) and they are three different colors of apples, twelve cherries, one nectarine, one mango, one slice of pineapple, one slice of cantaloupe, eight green grapes, one apricot, and one peach. In addition I also, eat eight raw Brazil nuts, 6 apricot nuts, one teaspoon of sunflower seeds, and one teaspoon of pumpkin seeds, two capsules of calcium, two capsules of magnesium.

For dinner, I usually have a salad, which consists of red or green head lettuce three radishes cut small one long green, onion cut small one third of a carrot, cut small one-half of avocado one-half of celery stalk cut small six tablespoons of lemon juice approximately one tablespoon or more of Braggs Ammino up to twelve ounces or more of two different kinds of Hot Sauce bread, or crackers, or corn tortillas Please do not copy or give away any material, not just, because it is copyright protected material, but doing this will interfere with my program of feeding and educating the unhealthy. All book proceeds as of 2008 have gone into this program. Instead my wish is that you do share your cooking with friends, family, and strangers.

Questions, concerns, and suggestions are welcome:

7619 N "8th" St
Fresno, CA 93720-2644
Phone 559 435 4069

14 DAYS OF MEALS

Day 1

Dinner: Salad, crackers, stuffed Bell peppers.

Dessert: Walnut Pie

Breakfast: Raw nut mix, fruit, toast with apricot jam

Day 2

Dinner: Salad, garlic bread, lentils and rice

Dessert: Orange macaroons

Breakfast: Raw nut mix, fruit, pumpkin seed waffles

Day 3

Dinner: Salad, corn tortillas, egg rolls

Dessert: Pineapple ice cream

Breakfast: Raw nut mix, fruit, cajon dry roasted nut mix

Day 4

Dinner: Tostadas, Lavash- tonir bread

Dessert: Lemon ice cream

Breakfast: Raw nut mix, fruit, pancakes

Day 5

Dinner: Salad, crackers, pot pie

Dessert: Pecan candy

Breakfast: Raw nut mix, fruit, Cajun rice

Day 6

Dinner: Salad, Lavash- tonir bread, spicy twice baked potatoes, jamaican rice

Dessert: Orange baked alaska

Breakfast: Raw nut mix, fruit, habanero lemon rice

Day 7

Dinner: Salad, corn tortillas, pocket pizzas

Dessert: Carob coconut cookies

Breakfast: Raw nut mix, fruit, bell pepper rice mix

Day 8

Dinner: Salad, Lavash-tonir bread, pasta

Dessert: Vanilla donuts

Breakfast: Raw nut mix, fruit, garlic and herbs baked rice

Day 9

Dinner: Salad, chinese rice, pan fried noodles, garlic bread

Dessert: Peppermint salt water taffy

Breakfast: Raw nut mix, fruit, cashew waffles

Day 10

Dinner: Salad, crackers, vegetable soup

Dessert: Peach cream pie

Breakfast: Raw nut mix, fruit, walnut waffles

Day 11

Dinner: Salad, cornbread, black eyed peas with rice

Dessert: Licorice Ice cream

Breakfast: Raw nut mix, fruit, popcorn

Day 12

Dinner: Salad, Lavash- tonir bread, tamale bean casserole

Dessert: Date tofu cookies

Breakfast: Raw nut mix, fruit, toast with almond butter

Day 13

Dinner: Salad, Lavash-tonir bread, potato and cabbage stew

Dessert: Plum cup cookies

Breakfast: Raw nut mix, fruit, toast with cherry jam

Day 14

Dinner: Salad, crackers, enchiladas

Dessert: Carob pie

Breakfast: Raw nut mix, fruit, green pepper rice

Recipe 544

Lemon and DILL Dry Roasted Nut Mix

Place the following and mix in a large bowl:

4 cups of walnuts

4 cups of pecans

4 cups of almonds

Spray with Braggs until all nuts are wet.

Mix and add:

One half cup of lemon powder

1 tablespoon of biosalt

2 to 4 tablespoons of Dill

Mix and spray again with Braggs.

Mix and add:

3 cups of Puffed corn or puffed rice

Spray again with Braggs until all ingredients are wet,

Place on tray lined with cookie mat.

Bake 200 degrees 12 hours or more until crisp.

Recipe 545

Lemon and Salted Dry Roasted Nut Mix

Place the following and mix in a large bowl:

4 cups of walnuts

4 cups of pecans

4 cups of almonds

Spray with Braggs until all nuts are wet.

Mix and add:

One half cup of lemon powder

1 tablespoon of biosalt

Mix and spray again with Braggs.

Mix and add:

3 cups of Puffed corn or puffed rice

Spray again with Braggs until all ingredients are wet,

Place on tray lined with cookie mat.

Bake 200 degrees 12 hours or more until crisp.

Recipe 546

Sweet and sour Dry Roasted Nut Mix

Place the following and mix in a large bowl:

4 cups of walnuts

4 cups of pecans

4 cups of almonds

Spray with Braggs until all nuts are wet.

Mix and add:

One to one half cup of lemon powder

2 cups of sucanat sugar

1 tablespoon of biosalt

Mix and spray again with Braggs.

Mix and add:

3 cups of Puffed corn or puffed rice

Spray again with Braggs until all ingredients are wet,

Place on tray lined with cookie mat.

Bake 200 degrees 12 hours or more until crisp.

Recipe 547

Lemon and Cayenne Dry Roasted Nut Mix

Place the following and mix in a large bowl:

4 cups of walnuts

4 cups of pecans

4 cups of almonds

Spray with Braggs until all nuts are wet.

Mix and add:

one half cup of lemon powder

3 to 5 tablespoons of cayenne powder

1 tablespoon of biosalt

Mix and spray again with Braggs.

Mix and add:

3 cups of Puffed corn or puffed rice

Spray again with Braggs until all ingredients are wet,

Place on tray lined with cookie mat.

Bake 200 degrees 12 hours or more until crisp.

Recipe 548

Lemon and Cajun Dry Roasted Nut Mix

Place the following in a large bowl:

4 cups of walnuts

4 cups of pecans

4 cups of almonds

Mix and lightly Spray with Braggs until all nuts are wet.

Mix and add:

one half cup of lemon powder

1 tablespoon of biosalt

1 tablespoon of garlic powder

1 tablespoon of onion powder

1 tablespoon of paprika powder

1 tablespoon of chili powder

spray again with Braggs.

Mix and add:

3 cups of Puffed corn or puffed rice

Spray again with Braggs until all ingredients are wet,

Place on tray lined with cookie mat.

Bake 200 degrees 12 hours or more until crisp.

Recipe 549

Lemon and Habanero Dry Roasted Nut Mix

Place the following in a large bowl: and mix:

4 cups of walnuts

4 cups of pecans

4 cups of almonds

lightly Spray all nuts with Braggs until wet. then mix and add (place this into vitamix)

12 Habanero peppers

one third cup of maple syrup

one fourth cup of braggs

Pour into nut mix.

mix and add:

1 tablespoon of biosalt

one half cup of lemon powder

Mix and spray again with Braggs. until all ingredients are wet.

add:

3 cups of Puffed corn or puffed rice

Mix and Spray again with Braggs until all ingredients are wet,

Place on tray lined with cookie mat.

Bake 200 degrees 12 hours or more until crisp.

Recipe 550

Lemon & Onion Dry Mix

Place the following in a large bowl: and mix:

4 cups of walnuts

4 cups of pecans

4 cups of almonds

lightly Spray all nuts with Braggs until wet. then mix and add (place this into
   vitamix)

12 Habanero peppers

one third cup of maple syrup

one fourth cup of braggs

Pour into nut mix.

mix and add:

1 tablespoon of biosalt

one half cup of lemon powder

2 tablespoons Onion powder

Mix and spray again with Braggs. until all ingredients are wet.

add:

3 cups of Puffed corn or puffed rice

Mix and Spray again with Braggs until all ingredients are wet,

Place on tray lined with cookie mat.

Bake 200 degrees 12 hours or more until crisp.

Recipe 551

Lemon and Garlic Dry Roasted Nut Mix

Place the following in a large bowl: and mix:

4 cups of walnuts

4 cups of pecans

4 cups of almonds

Mix and lightly Spray all nuts with Braggs until wet.

ADD:

1 Tablespoon of biosalt

one half cup of lemon powder

2 tablespoons of garlic powder

Mix and spray again with Braggs. until all ingredients are wet.

add:

3 cups of Puffed corn or puffed rice

Mix and Spray again with Braggs until all ingredients are wet,

Place on tray lined with cookie mat.

Bake 200 degrees 12 hours or more until crisp.

Recipe 552

NECTARINE ICE CREAM

Place all of the following into a vitamix and blend until smooth

2 cups of a Agave Nectar

3 cups of puffed rice

1 c pitted nectarines

2c walnuts

¼ tsp biosalt

½ - 1 cup almond milk

1 brick or 1 lb. tofu

1 tablespoon almond butter

Pour into ½ pint jars and freeze

SPICE ICE CREAM

Place all of the following into a vitamix and blend until smooth

2 cups of a Agave Nectar

3 cups of puffed rice

2c walnuts

¼ tsp biosalt

½ - 1 cup almond milk

1 tablespoon almond butter

½ - 1 tsp cinnamon

¼ - ½ tsp clove powder

½ - 1 tsp ginger powder

1 brick or 1 lb. tofu

Pour into ½ pint jars and freeze

Recipe 554

THIN CORN BREAD

Place into vitamix all of the following:

1c whole wheat pastry flour

1c cornmeal or corn flour

½ tsp biosalt

1 tsp cayenne powder

2 tsp agave nectar

¼ c tofu

1¼ c almond milk

blend until smooth

spread thin on cookie tray with lined cookie mat

bake 10 minutes 425 degrees

yield: 1 recipe per tray

Recipe 555

NECTARINE CREAM PIE

Crust: see recipe number 38

place into vitamix 5 lbs. pitted nectarines

do not add water

add the following:

1 c agave nectar

1c succrant sugar

1 large apple remove core only

Blend until smooth, pour into a large container

bring to boil and simmer on warm for 1 hour or until thick

Stir occasionally

Pour mixture into 2 pie shells, extra mixture can freeze

Place top crumb crust (no agave syrup)

Bake 45 minutes 350 degrees, Cool

Recipe 556

CINNAMON PIE

Crust: see recipe number 38

Mix in a large bowl the following:

1c sucanant sugar

1/2c almond butter

3 tablespoons cinnamon powder

1 tsp vanilla

1/2c tofu

Mix and add 2c chopped walnuts

mix thoroughly and pour into pie shell level and

pour 1c agave nectar on top of pie

Bake 25 minutes at 375 degrees

Cool for 2 hrs in refrigerator

Recipe 557

CINNAMON CHEESECAKE

Crust: see recipe number 38 (no added agave nectar)

mix into a 10x10 springform 3 inches deep

Place the following into a vitamix:

2c tofu

3 tablespoon cinnamon powder

1c almond milk

1 tablespoon vanilla

1/4 c whole wheat pastry flour

11/2 c sucanat sugar

Mix and pour into pan

bake 325 degrees about 1 hour 15 min

Cool and refrigerate 2-3 hours

Recipe 558

CINNAMON DATE PASTRY

Crust:

Mix in a large bowl the following:

2c agave nectar

1c chopped walnuts

1/3 c Carob powder

1/3c cinnamon

2c almond butter

set aside 2 cups mixture

pour into a lined 1 inch cookie tray

Filling

Mix in a large bowl the following:

2c of above mixture

1c chopped walnuts

2c agave nectar

3c dates chopped small

Mix and add to pie crust

Bake 350 at 20 minutes

Glaze:

Mix and add

1c agaur nectua

2 tablespoon cinnamon

1/4c carob powder

Spread on top and refrigerate

Recipe 559

CARAMELIZED CINNAMON TART

Crust:

Mix in a large bowl the following:

1c almond butter

4 tablespoons agave nectar

¼ tsp biosalt

1 tsp vanilla

2c sifted whole wheat pastry flour

Mix and place, form into a 12x7 in round pan lined with parchment paper

filling:

Mix in a large pan the following: bring to a boil then 10 minutes on low

3c agave nectar

1/2c carob powder

4c chopped walnuts

3 tablespoon cinnamon powder

1/2c dates chopped small

Mix and pour into baked crust

Bake 8 minutes at 400 degrees

cool and refrigerate 2-4 hours

Recipe 560

CINNAMON CANDY

Place the following in a large pan Boil on low for 30 minutes:

3 tablespoon almond milk

1 tsp bio salt

6 tablespoons almond butter

6 c maple syrup

Stir occasionally; Add

6 tablespoons cinnamon Boil 15 minutes
.

Add:

3c chopped walnuts and and Boil 15 minutes

Add

3c puffed rice and Boil 15 minutes

Mix and Stir Continually to boil until mixture is thick

Pour thick mixture on parchment papers spread evenly and cover mixture with parchment paper

Roll with rolling pins until thin layer, let cool and break into desired shapes, place into plastic bags and store in refrigerator

Recipe 561

LICORICE ICE CREAM

Place the following ingredients into vitamix and Blend until smooth:

¼-½ tsp liquid anise

¼ tsp biosalt

3c puffed rice

2c walnuts

1 tablespoonful almond butter

2c agave nectar

½-1c almond milk

1 brick or 1 lb tofu

After mixed, pour into 6 ounce jars and freeze

LICORICE FROSTING

Place 6c sucrant sugar into vitamix using 2 cups at a time and blend into powder

Pour into a large bowl and add the following:

3 tablespoon agave nectar

¼-½ tsp liquid anise

For thinner frosting add water or almond milk 1 tablespoon at a time

Place on cool cake, refrigerate until frosting sets

Recipe 563

LICORICE BAKED ALASKA

Place the following into vitamix

1c sucanat sugar

1c agave nectar

1c almond butter

1 brick or 1 lb tofu

¼-½ tsp. liquid anise

blend until all ingredients are smooth

Pour into 4-5 mini oven cups

Bake 350 degrees 20 minutes

LICORICE CHEESE CAKE

Crust: see recipe number 38 (no added agave nectar)

mix into a 10x10 springform 3 inches deep

Place the following into a vitamix:

2c tofu

¼-½ tsp liquid anise

1c almond milk

1 tablespoon vanilla

1/4 c whole wheat pastry flour

11/2 c sucanat sugar

Mix and pour into pan

bake 325 degrees about 1 hour 15 min

Cool and refrigerate 2-3 hours

Recipe 565

LICORICE TOFFEE COOKIE

Mix in a bowl the following:

¼-1/2 tsp liquid anise

1c almond butter

1c sucanat sugar

1/4c tofu

Mix and add 2c Sifted whole wheat flour

Mix and place into a 9x9 lined cake pan

level and press mixture and ADD 1c chopped walnuts press into mixture

bake 1 hour at 275 degrees Cool

Recipe 566

LICORICE FUDGE

Boil and bring to warm for 5 minutes

2 1/2c sucanat sugar

1c maple syrup

Boil additional 5 minutes and Add

¼-1/2 tsp liquid anise

Boil additional 5 minutes and Add

2c chopped walnuts

Mix and boil 5 more minutes Add

2c almond butter

Pour into 8x8 glass baking dish, lined with parchment paper

Press mixture cool and refrigerate 2 hrs until firm

Recipe 567

LICORICE SALT WATER TOFFEE

Place in a small pan and boil for 30 minutes on warm:

1c sucanat sugar

1c maple syrup

¼-½ tsp liquid anise

½ tsp biosalt

1/2c water

2 tablespoon cornstarch

2 tablespoon almond butter

Continue to boil and mix, check Freezer test before removing from heat

place a few drops of mixture on dish place into freezer for 30 seconds

if mixture soft repeat freezer test, when firm then Add

2 tsp vanilla do not stir let set for 10 minutes.

spread on cookie mat and cool

break into bite size shapes and wrap in wax paper.

store in refrigerator

Recipe 568

LICORICE COCONUT CARAMELS

Place the following into vitamix for 5 min:

1c maple syrup

1c almond milk

2 tsp vanilla

¼-½ tsp liquid anise

1 tsp biosalt

1 ½ c sucanat sugar

1 large or 2 small apples

Then pour into a medium size pan and bow on low for 50-60 minutes

Stir occasionally

lined a 8x8 glass dish lined with parchment paper

Add 1c dried coconut flour inside dish and set aside

Start Freezer test 45 minutes into boiling

Freezer test, place in a small dish 1 spoon of mixture put in freezer for 1 minute
    check for firmness

at 55 minutes into boiling repeat freezer test, check firmness at 60 minutes mixture should be done

Pour into 8x8 dish

Place in refrigerator uncovered for 24 hours then cut into bite size squares and wrap in wax paper stored in refrigerator

LICORICE CANDY

Place the following in a large pan Boil on low for 30 minutes:

3 tablespoon almond milk

1 tsp bio salt

6 tablespoons almond butter

6 c maple syrup

Stir occasionally; Add

¼- ½ tsp liquid anaise Boil 15 minutes

Add:

3c chopped walnuts and and Boil 15 minutes

Add

3c puffed rice and Boil 15 minutes

Mix and Stir Continually to boil until mixture is thick

Pour thick mixture on parchment papers spread evenly and cover mixture with parchment paper

Roll with rolling pins until thin layer, let cool and break into desired shapes, place into plastic bags and store in refrigerator

LICORICE COCONUT COOKIES

Mix the following in a large bowl:

6c maple syrup

1 tsp biosalt

2c oatmeal flour

4c coconut flour

¼ -½ tsp liquid anise

Add 5c sifted whole wheat pastry flour

Form cookies on trays lined with cookie mat

Bake 325 degrees for 25 minutes

Recipe 571

LICORICE MACARONS

Place the following into vitamix:

1c apple

2c maple syrup

2c sucanat sugar

2c almond butter

2 tsp vanilla

1 tsp biosalt

¼-/2 tsp liquid anise

Pour into a large bowl

Add 5c sifted whole wheat pastry flour

Form cookies on tray lined with cookie mat

Bake 375 degrees for 15 minutes

Mix dough 24 hours ahead and refrigerate

Recipe 572

HAVANERO RICE

Place in large pan the following: Day before

8c water

6c rice

1 tsp biosalt

Day 2 bring to a boil then low for 10-15 minutes, add lid

Place the following into vitamix Blend until smooth:

1 tablespoon chile powder

1 tablespoon paprika

1 tablespoon biosalt

1 tablespoon garlic powder

1 tablespoon onion powder

1c cilantro

12-15 habanero peppers

1/2c lemon juice

Add to rice and mix, turn stove off, leave lid for 10-15 minutes

Recipe 573

MARTIN MASSOOD LICORICE SANDWICH COOKIES

Place the following into vitamix:

½-1 tsp liquid anise

2c maple syrup

½ sucrose sugar

4c pitted dates

¼ tsp biosalt

1 tsp water

Blend until smooth, pour into large covered bowl and refrigerate Day before

in another bowl Add 2c chopped walnuts cover bowl place in refrigerator

For Dough see recipe number 45

next day roll out dough using rolling pin roll into thin layer

using a round 3x3 inch cookie cutter cut into dough circles, place 1 -2 spoons of
   mixture into cookie

Add 1-2 tsp walnuts on top Place second cookie circle on top and press together to form a sandwich

Place on trays lined with cookie mat using a plastic fork press down tops of cookies twice

Bake 325 degrees 15-20 minutes

Recipe 574

CINNAMON SANDWICH COOKIES

Place the following into vitamix blend until smooth:

2c maple syrup

1-3 tablespoon cinnamon powder

½ c sucanat sugar

4c pitted dates

¼ tsp biosalt

1 tsp water

Blend until smooth, pour into large covered bowl and refrigerate Day before

in another bowl Add 2c chopped walnuts cover bowl place in refrigerator

For Dough see recipe number 45

next day roll out dough using rolling pin roll into thin layer

using a round 3x3 inch cookie cutter cut into dough circles, place 1 -2 spoons of
mixture into cookie

Add 1-2 tsp walnuts on top Place second cookie circle on top and press together to form a sandwich

Place on trays lined with cookie mat using a plastic fork press down tops of cookies twice

Bake 325 degrees 15-20 minutes

Recipe 575

CORN ON THE COB

Place cleaned corn in a large pan covered with water

bring to a boil then lower 5-10 minutes until cooked

drain water and serve hot

Spray corn with Braggs Amino and can add lemon juice for taste

Sprinkle italian seasoning for taste

AVA DANIELLE NEUMILLER ORANGE CREAM PIE

Place the following into vitamix:

1 brick or 1 lb tofu

1c maple syrup

1c almond butter

1c sucanat sugar

1/2 c whole wheat pastry flour

1/4c orange rind or powder

3 tablespoon orange juice

Blend until smooth pour into unbaked pie shell (see recipe 38)

Bake 350 degrees for 20 minutes

Serve chilled

Recipe 577

CINNAMON WALNUT FUDGE

Boil and bring to warm for 5 minutes

2 1/2c sucanat sugar

1c maple syrup

Boil additional 5 minutes and Add

1-2 tsp cinnamon powder

Boil additional 5 minutes and Add

2c chopped walnuts

Mix and boil 5 more minutes Add

2c almond butter

Pour into 8x8 glass baking dish, lined with parchment paper

Press mixture cool and refrigerate 2 hrs until firm

Recipe 578

WALNUT CRUST FOR ANY PIE

Place the following into vitamix:

1c walnuts

1c oatmeal

1/4c coconut

1/4 tsp biosalt

Mix and blend until smooth and pour into pie dish

Add 3 tablespoon maple syrup and mix

Form into pie shell,

Add filling

Bake 350 degrees 45 minutes (fruit pies add top crumb crust No maple syrup)

when using top crusts, yields 2 pies

Recipe 579

GREEN PEAS AND RICE

Day before in a large pan and set aside

Place 6c rice

8c water

tablespoon biosalt

day two in small pan

2 lbs green peas

6 tablespoon lemon juice

3 tablespoon Braggs Amino

1c chopped small cilantro

Boil on low 5-10 minutes when done aside

Bring rice to boil turn to low Place lid on pan let set

Add pea mixture and stir into rice and stir, let set and serve

LEMON CREAM PIE

Place the following into a vitamix and Blend until smooth:

1 lb or 1 brick tofu

1c maple syrup

1c sucanat sugar

1c almond butter

½c whole wheat pastry flour

1/4c lemon rind

2 tablespoon lemon powder

After mix and smooth pour into unbaked pie shell

Bake 350 degrees 20 minutes cool

Place in refrigerator for 2 hours served chilled

Recipe 581

COCONUT CREAM PIE

Place the following into a vitamix and Blend until smooth:

1 lb or 1 brick tofu

1c maple syrup

1c sucanant sugar

1c almond butter

½c whole wheat pastry flour

2c coconut flour

3 tablespoon pineapple juice

After mix and smooth pour into unbaked pie shell

Bake 350 degrees 20 minutes cool

Place in refrigerator for 2 hours served chilled

PUMPKIN AND APPLE COOKIES

Place into vitamix 2 1/2c oatmeal and make into a flour

Pour into a large bowl with 4c sifted whole wheat pastry flour, set aside

Place the following into a vitamix

1/2c tofu

2 tablespoons vanilla

2c pumpkin

1/2c almond butter

1 tsp ginger powder

½ tsp clove powder

1 tsp biosalt

4 tsp cinnamon powder

1 large or 2 small apples

Blend until smooth, pour into above large bowl and mix

Add 2c sucanat sugar and mix

Form cookies on trays lined with cookie mat

Bake 325 degrees 25 minutes

Recipe 583

SUCANANT FACE COOKIES

Place the following in a large bowl and mix.

1 Cup of maple syrup

2 teaspoons of biosalt

4 tablespoons of soy milk

1 cup of tofu

4 teaspoons of vanilla

Mix well and add

4 cups of sucanant sugar

3 cups of almond butter

2 cups of oatmeal flour

3 cups of Whole wheat pastry flour (sifted)

Mix well and roll into balls, approximate size One and one half to 2 inches.

dip - press balls into bowl of sucanant sugar

one side only. Cookie ball will flatten into a circle.

Place on trays lined with cookie mat, 9 per tray

Bake 325 degrees 25 minutes

Recipe 584

HAZELNUT FACE COOKIES

Place the following in a large bowl and mix.

1 Cup of maple syrup

2 teaspoons of biosalt

4 tablespoons of soy milk

1 cup of tofu

4 teaspoons of vanilla

Mix well and add

4 cups of sucanant sugar

3 cups of almond butter

2 cups of oatmeal flour

3 cups of Whole wheat pastry flour (sifted)

Mix well and roll into balls, approximate size One and one half to 2 inches.

dip - press into bowl of chopped Hazelnuts (approximately 2 - 3 cups)----

one side only. Cookie ball will flatten into a circle.

Place on trays lined with cookie mat, 9 per tray

Bake 325 degrees 25 minutes

Recipe 585

HAZELNUT CAROB COOKIES

Place the following in a large bowl and mix.

1 Cup of maple syrup

2 teaspoons of biosalt

4 teaspoons of vanilla

1 cup of Tofu

One fourth cup of carob

Mix and add

4 cups of sucanant sugar

3 cups of almond butter

2 cups of oatmeal flour

3 cups of Whole wheat pastry flour (sifted)

Mix and roll into balls, Size One and one half to 2 inches

dip - press into bowl of chopped Hazel nuts (approximately 2 - 3 cups)

one side only. balls will flatten into a circle.

Place on trays lined with cookie mat 9 per tray

Bake 325 degrees 25 minutes

Recipe 586

PISTACHIO FACE COOKIES

Place the following in a large bowl and mix.

1 Cup of maple syrup

2 teaspoons of biosalt

4 tablespoons of soy milk

1 cup of tofu

4 teaspoons of vanilla

Mix well and add

4 cups of sucanant sugar

3 cups of almond butter

2 cups of oatmeal flour

3 cups of Whole wheat pastry flour (sifted)

Mix well and roll into balls, approximate size One and one half to 2 inches.

dip - press into bowl of chopped Pistachios (approximately 2 - 3 cups)----

one side only. Cookie ball will flatten into a circle.

Place on trays lined with cookie mat, 9 per tray

Bake 325 degrees 25 minutes

Recipe 587

PILAF RICE MIX

Place in a large pan the following: Day before mix and set aside

6c rice

2 tsp biosalt

7c water

next day add into pan

1c shredded carrot

1 tsp rosemary

1c slivered almonds

12 ounces any pasta or pizza sauce

1 chopped onion

1/2c almond butter

Bring to a boil lower for 10-15 minutes as needed add lid add water as needed

PERO SUCANANT COOKIES

Place the following into large bowl and mix:

1 Cup of maple syrup

1 Cup of tofu

2 teaspoons of biosalt

4 teaspoons of vanilla

One fourth cup of Pero - Natural Coffee

Mix and add the following:

4 cups of sucanant sugar

3 cups of almond butter

2 cups of oatmeal flour

3 cups of Whole wheat pastry flour (sifted)

Mix and roll into balls, approximate size One and one half to 2 inches.

dip - press balls into a bowl of sucanant sugar

one side only.

Ball will flatten into a circle.

Place on trays lined with cookie mat, 9 per tray

Bake 325 degrees 25 minutes

Recipe 589

HAZELNUT SPICE COOKIES

Place the following into large bowl and mix:

1 Cup of maple syrup

1 Teaspoon of ginger

1 teaspoon of clove powder

1 teaspoon of cinnamon

2 teaspoons of biosalt

4 tablespoons of soy milk

1 cup of tofu

4 teaspoons of vanilla

Mix and add the following:

4 cups of sucanant sugar

3 cups of almond butter

2 cups of oatmeal flour

3 cups of Whole wheat pastry flour (sifted)

Mix well and roll into balls, approximate size One and one half to 2 inches.

dip - press into a bowl of chopped

Hazel nuts (approximately 2 - 3 cups)

one side only.

Cookie balls will flatten into a circle.

Place on trays lined with cookie mat, 9 per tray

Bake 325 degrees 25 minutes

Let Cool. Can freeze extra.

CINNAMON WALNUT FACE COOKIES

Place the following into large bowl and mix:

1 Cup of maple syrup

2 teaspoons of biosalt

4 tablespoons of soy milk

1 cup of tofu

4 teaspoons of vanilla

2- 3 tablespoons cinnamon

Mix and add :

4 cups of sucanant sugar

3 cups of almond butter

2 cups of oatmeal flour

3 cups of Whole wheat pastry flour (sifted)

Mix well and roll into balls, approximate size One and one half to 2 inches.

dip - press into a bowl of chopped

Walnuts (approximately 2 - 3 cups)

one side only.

Cookie balls will flatten into a circle.

Place on trays lined with cookie mat, 9 per tray

Bake 325 degrees 25 minutes

Recipe 591

Carob-coconut Face Cookies

Place the following into a large bowl and mix:

One cup of maple syrup

Two teaspoons of Biosalt

Four tablespoons of soy milk

Four teaspoons of vanilla

One cup of tofu

One fourth cup of carob

Mix and add:

Four cups of sucanat sugar

Three cups of almond butter

Three cups of whole wheat pastry flour (sifted)

Two cups of oatmeal flour

Mix and roll into balls approximately size one and one half to two

inches. Dip – press into bowl of Coconut Lite (powder) one side only – cookie ball
will flatten into a circle.

Place on trays lined with cookie mat. 9 per tray.

Bake 325 degrees 25 minutes

Recipe 592

LEMON WALNUT COOKIES

Place the following in a large bowl and mix:

One cup of maple syrup

One cup of Tofu

One cup of lemon rind

One tablespoon of soy milk

Four teaspoons of vanilla

Two teaspoons of biosalt

Mix and add:

Four cups of sucanat sugar

Three cups of almond butter

Three cups whole wheat pastry flour

Two cups of oatmeal flour

Mix and roll into balls approximately one and a half inches by two inches. Dip – press into a bowl of chopped walnuts (approximately 2 – 3 cups) one side only. Cookie ball will flatten into circle. Place on trays lined with cookie mat. 9 per tray.

Bake 325 degrees 25 minutes

Recipe 593

ORANGE WALNUT COOKIES

Place following into large bowl and mix;

One cup of maple syrup

One cup of tofu

One cup of orange rind

Four tablespoons of soy milk

Two teaspoons of biosalt

Four teaspoons of vanilla

Mix and add:

Four cups of sucanant sugar

Three cups of almond butter

Two cups of oatmeal flour

Three cups of whole wheat pastry flour (sifted)

Mix well and roll into balls one and one half inches – two inches.

Dip – press into bowl of chopped walnuts (two – three cups) –one side Only. Cookie balls will flatten into a circle. Place on trays lined with

Cookie mat. Nine per tray.

Bake 325 degrees 25 minutes

Recipe 594

ANISE WALNUT COOKIES

Place following into large bowl and mix:

one cup of maple syrup

one cup of tofu

Four tablespoons of soy milk

Two teaspoons of biosalt

Four teaspoons of vanilla

One half or one and a half teaspoons of liquid Anise, this depends on how strong of a licorice taste you desire. Always start with one half teaspoon on your first recipe.

Mix well and add:

Four cups of sucanat sugar

Three cups of almond butter

Three cups of whole wheat pastry flour (sifted)

Two cups of oatmeal flour

Mix well and roll into balls – one and one half to two inches, dip – press balls into a bowl of chopped walnuts (2 – 3 cups) one side only. Cookies will flatten into a circle. Place on trays lined with cookie mat. 9 per tray.

Bake 325 degrees 25 minutes

Recipe 595

PEPPERMINT WALNUT COOKIES

Place into a large bowl the following and mix:

1 cup of Maple syrup

1 cup of tofu

Four teaspoons of vanilla

Two teaspoons of Biosalt

One fourth or one half or one teaspoon of peppermint liquid.

This depends on how strong a peppermint taste you desire.

Always start with one fourth teaspoon on your first recipe.

Mix well and add:

Four cups of sucanant sugar

Three cups of almond butter

Two cups of oatmeal flour

Three cups of whole wheat pastry flour (sifted)

Mix well and roll into balls one and one half inches – two inches.

Dip and press into bowl of chopped walnuts (two – three cups) one side only. Cookie balls will flatten into a circle. Place on trays lined with cookie mat.

Bake 325 degrees 25 minutes

Recipe 596

CAROB COCONUT PIE COOKIES

Mix in a large bowl the following:

One cup of almond butter

Two cups of sucanant sugar

One fourth cup of tofu

One fourth cup of Carob

Mix and add:

Two cups of whole wheat pastry flour (sifted)

Mix again and place into a 9 X 9 inch cake pan lined with Parchment paper.

Press into pan with back side of spoon.

Place one cup of Coconut Lite on top and press into dough.

Bake 275 degrees One hour

Let cool -- cut into pie shapes 16 parts

Recipe 597

PERO AND HAZELNUT PIE COOKIES

Mix in a large bowl the following:

Two cups of sucanant sugar

One cup of Almond Butter

One fourth cup of Tofu

One cup of Pero – not coffee

Mix and add:

Two cups of whole wheat pastry flour (sifted)

Mix again and place into a 9 x 9 inch cake pan lined with Parchment paper.

Press into pan with back side of a spoon. Add one cup of chopped Hazelnuts on top of pan and press into dough.

Bake 275 degrees for 1 hour

Let cool -- cut into pie shapes 16 parts.

Recipe 598

CARAMELIZED CINNAMON PISTACHIO TART

Place in a large bowl and mix the following:

(CRUST)

One cup of almond butter

Four tablespoons of maple syrup

One fourth teaspoon of Biosalt

One teaspoon of vanilla

Two cups of whole wheat pastry flour (sifted)

Place in a pan 12 x 7 inches lined with parchment paper.

Bake 10 minutes at 350 degrees.

Set aside.

(Filling) Boil in a pan for 10 minutes on low the following:

Three cups of maple syrup

One half cup dried pineapple or papaya or dates chopped.

Four teaspoons of cinnamon

One half cup of carob

Four cups of chopped Pistachios

Add to boiled custard, return to oven for 8 minutes at 400 degrees.

Recipe 599

VITAMIX LICORICE MACARONS

Place the following into large bowl:

One hundred roasted chopped almonds

One and a half cups of any dried chopped fruit

One fourth to one half teaspoons of liquid Anise

Set aside

Place in Vitamix nine cups of coconut

Blend until becomes liquified.

Pour and mix into the above large bowl. Form cookies on trays lined with cookie
    mat, then place in refrigerator to harden. Serve cold.

Recipe 600

VITAMIX CINNAMON MACAROONS

Place following into a large bowl:

One hundred roasted and chopped almonds.

One and a half cups of any dried fruit chopped.

One to two tablespoons of cinnamon this depends on your desired taste.

Mix and set aside.

Place in a vitamix nine cups of coconut

Blend until it becomes liquified.

Pour and mix into the above bowl.

Form cookies on trays lined with cookie mat then place in refrigerator to harden.

Serve cold.

Recipe 601

VITAMIX PEPPERMINT MACARONS

Place the following into a large bowl:

Two cups of chopped walnuts

One fourth or one half teaspoon of liquid peppermint

This depends on your taste always start with one fourth teaspoon on our first recipe.

One and one half cups of any dry fruit chopped.

Mix and set aside.

Place into VITAMIX 9 cups of coconut

Blend until coconut becomes liquefied.

Pour into the above large bowl and mix.

Form cookies on trays lined with cookie mat.

Place in refrigerator to harden,

Serve cold.

Recipe 602

WINTINSON STRAWBERRY CREAM PIE

For pie crust see recipe # 38

Place into VITAMIX one and one half pounds of fresh and clean Strawberries.

DO NOT ADD ANY WATER, and add the following:

One cup of maple syrup

One cup of sucanant sugar

Two large apples or four small apples (remove core only)

One fourth teaspoon of biosalt

Blend until smooth and pour into large pan and boil on warm for one hour. Mixture will become thicker. Pour into pie shell, place top crust,

(However do not add any maple syrup) this is a crumb crust, cover pie.

Helpful Hint: Top crust is enough for two pies.

Bake 350 degrees 45 minutes

Recipe 603

STRAWBERRY ICE CREAM

Place all these ingredients into VITAMIX and blend until smooth:

One fourth teaspoon of biosalt

Two cups of maple syrup

One tablespoon of almond butter

Two – three cups of strawberries

Three cups of Puffed Rice

Two cups of walnuts

One brick or one pound of tofu

One half -one cup of soymilk

Continue to mix until all ingredients are smooth, pour into six ounce jars and place
into freezer.

Recipe 604

STRAWBERRY CHEESECAKE

(CRUST) Make crust first. See special pie crust recipe #38

DO NOT ADD ANY MAPLE SYRUP.

Mix and add crust to a springform pan 10 X 10 inches – three inches deep lined
with parchment paper -- set aside.

(FILLING)

Place the following into VITAMIX:

Two cups of tofu

One half cup of soymilk

One and one half cups of strawberries

One tablespoon of vanilla

One fourth cup of whole wheat pastry flour

One and one half cups of sucanant sugar

Pour into the above pan

Bake one hour and fifteen minutes at 325 degrees

Recipe 605

BLUEBERRY CHEESECAKE

(CRUST) --Make crust first

See special pie crust recipe#38

DO NOT ADD ANY MAPLE SYRUP

Mix and add crust to a springform pan 10 x 10 inches -- three inches deep, lined
with parchment paper – set aside.

(FILLING)

Place the following into a VITAMIX

Two cups of tofu

One half cup of soymilk

One and one half cups of Blueberries

One tablespoon of vanilla

One fourth cup of whole wheat pastry flour

One and one half cups of sucanant sugar

Pour into the above pan.

Bake one hour and fifteen minutes at 325 degrees.

Recipe 606

STRAWBERRY BAKED ALASKA

Place the following into VITAMIX:

One cup of sucanant sugar

One brick or one pound of tofu

One and one half cups of strawberries

One cup of almond butter

One cup of maple syrup

Mix until smooth, pour into baking dishes 7 x 7 inches – four or five needed.

Bake 350 degrees for 20 minutes.

Let cool.

Serve cold or semi frozen. Can freeze extra, covered.

STRAWBERRY MAPLE CAKE

Place into VITAMIX following:

Two cups cleaned strawberries

Two tablespoons of almond butter

One teaspoon of vanilla

One tablespoon of biosalt

Six cups of maple syrup

Mix and pour into large bowl and add:

Six cups of chopped walnuts

Four cups of sifted whole wheat pastry flour

Mix and pour into 13 x 9 inch glass dish, lined with parchment paper.

Bake 350 degrees for one and one half hours and after one hour use toothpick test
   to see if center is baked.

Let cake cool then cut.

Recipe 608

STRAWBERRY UPSIDE DOWN CREAM CAKE

(Mix dough first)

Place in VITAMIX the following:

Twelve tablespoons of Pineapple juice

Two cups of maple syrup

Two cups of almond butter

Mix and pour into large bowl with the following:

Six cups of whole wheat pastry flour (sifted)

Add yeast – follow yeast instructions or place two tablespoons of yeast into one half cup of finger warm water and mix. Pour into the above bowl and let sit for 30 minutes in a warm place covered -- dough should rise. Set aside.

(Topping) Line a round cake pan 10 x 10 inches with parchment paper at least three inches deep. Pour two cups of sucanant sugar and spread evenly. Next place one and one half pounds of cleaned strawberries and add one cup of maple syrup, and blend until smooth. Then pour into pan and add the above dough, spread evenly.

Bake 350 degrees 45 – 60 minutes or until baked

Use toothpick test to see if center is baked. Let cool for 30 minutes and place a large glass dish on top of pan and turn over.

Helpful Hint: Turn oven lower to prevent a boil or spill over, and can use a taller cake pan.

Recipe 609

FIRE DRY ROASTED NUT MIX

Place in a large bowl and mix:

Two cups of almonds

Four cups of walnuts

Four cups of pecans

Spray with BRAGGS until all nuts are covered.

Add six – eight tablespoons of cayenne pepper

(For first recipe start with four tablespoons)

Spray with BRAGGS and add one tablespoon of biosalt, and spray with BRAGGS and mix and add one tablespoon of paprika, and spray with BRAGGS and mix and add one tablespoon of chili powder, and mix and spray with BRAGGS, and add one tablespoon of onion powder, mix and spray BRAGGS and add one tablespoon of garlic powder, and mix and spray again with BRAGGS and add one half cup of powdered lemon, spray and mix with BRAGGS and add four cups of puffed corn and spray with BRAGGS and mix.

Place on one tray lined with cookie mat.

Bake 200 degrees for 12 – 15 hours overnight

Recipe 610

CITRUS AND HERB RICE

The night before soak six cups of rice.

One tablespoon of BIOSALT
Eight cups of water into a large pan. The next day bring to a boil, and then turn to
 low, for ten to fifteen minutes with lid on pan, until rice is cooked.

Add the following:

Mix and place lid on pan. Let sit for fifteen minutes or more. (turn off heat first)

Four tablespoons lemon rind
Four tablespoons of orange rind
One tablespoon of BIOSALT
One tablespoon of oregano
One tablespoon of onion powder
One tablespoon of garlic powder
One tablespoon of parsley
One teaspoon of basil

Serve hot and can freeze extra in one half quart jars.

Recipe 611

BARBECUE SEASONED RICE

The night before soak six cups of rice.

One tablespoon of BIOSALT
Eight cups of water Into a large pan,

The next day bring to a boil, and then turn to low for ten to fifteen minutes with
lid on, until rice is cooked.

Add the following:

Mix and place lid on pan fifteen minutes or more. (Turn heat off first)

Two tablespoons of paprika
Two tablespoons of red dry chili (flakes)
Three tablespoons of BRAGGS
One tablespoon of BIOSALT
Two tablespoons of cayenne
One tablespoon of nutmeg
One tablespoon of cumin
One tablespoon of onion powder

One tablespoon of garlic powder

Three tablespoons of lemon rind

Mix again, serve hot.

Can freeze extra in one half quart jars.

Recipe 612

MEXICAN SEASONED RICE

The night before soak six cups of rice.

One tablespoon of BIOSALT

Eight cups of water into large pan.

The next day bring to a boil and then turn to low for 10 -15 minutes.

Place lid on, until rice is cooked.

Add the following:

Mix and place lid on pan and let sit for 15 minutes or more, (turn off heat first)

Two tablespoons of Oregano
Four stalks of celery cut small
One tablespoon of cumin
One tablespoon of garlic powder
One tablespoon of BIOSALT
One tablespoon of paprika
One tablespoon of onion powder
One half quart of existing hot sauce

Serve hot -- can freeze extra in half quart jars.

Recipe 613

JAMAICAN SEASONED RICE

The night before soak six cups of rice.

One tablespoon of BIOSALT

Eight cups of water into large pan.

The next day bring to a boil and then turn to low for 10 -15 minutes.

Place lid on, until rice is cooked.

Add the following:

Mix and place lid on pan and let sit for 15 minutes or more, (turn off heat first)

One tablespoon of BIOSALT
One tablespoon of Ginger
One tablespoon of Cinnamon
One tablespoon of Maple syrup
One tablespoon of onion powder

One tablespoon of garlic powder

One half quart of existing hot sauce

Mix

Serve hot -- can freeze extra in half quart jars.

Recipe 614

ITALIAN SEASONED RICE

The night before soak six cups of rice.

One tablespoon of BIOSALT

Eight cups of water into large pan.

The next day bring to a boil and then turn to low for 10 -15 minutes.

Place lid on, until rice is cooked.

Add the following:

Mix and place lid on pan and let sit for 15 minutes or more, (turn off heat first)

Two tablespoons of Oregano
One tablespoon of BIOSALT
One teaspoon of Marjorm
One teaspoon of thyme
One teaspoon of rosemary

One teaspoon of sage

One teaspoon of basil

Mix

Serve hot -- can freeze extra in half quart jars.

TACO SEASONED RICE

The night before soak six cups of rice.

One tablespoon of BIOSALT

Eight cups of water into large pan.

The next day bring to a boil and then turn to low for 10 -15 minutes.

Place lid on, until rice is cooked.

Add the following:

Mix and place lid on pan and let sit for 15 minutes or more, (turn off heat first)

One tablespoon of chili powder
One tablespoon of onion powder
One tablespoon of garlic powder
One tablespoon of cumin
One tablespoon of paprika
One tablespoon of BIOSALT
One tablespoon of oregano
Three tablespoons of lemon rind

Two tablespoons of cornmeal

One half quart of existing hot sauce

Mix

Serve hot -- can freeze extra in half quart jars.

Recipe 616

THAI SEASONED RICE

The night before soak six cups of rice.

One tablespoon of BIOSALT

Eight cups of water into large pan.

The next day bring to a boil and then turn to low for 10 -15 minutes.

Place lid on, until rice is cooked.

Add the following:

Mix and place lid on pan and let sit for 15 minutes or more, (turn off heat first)

One tablespoon of basil
One tablespoon of paprika
Three tablespoons of lemon rind
One tablespoon of garlic powder
One tablespoon of onion powder
One tablespoon of coriander

One tablespoon of BIOSALT

One half quart of existing hot sauce

Mix

Serve hot -- can freeze extra in half quart jars.

Recipe 617

PIZZA SEASONED RICE

The night before soak six cups of rice.

One tablespoon of BIOSALT

Eight cups of water into large pan.

The next day bring to a boil and then turn to low for 10 -15 minutes.

Place lid on, until rice is cooked.

Add the following:

Mix and place lid on pan and let sit for 15 minutes or more, (turn off heat first)

One tablespoon of onion powder

One tablespoon of oregano

One tablespoon of garlic powder

One tablespoon of BIOSALT

One tablespoon of parsley

One teaspoon of MARJORAM

One teaspoon of thyme

One half quart of existing Pizza Sauce
Two Bell peppers cut small

(Boil with rice)

Mix again

Serve hot -- can freeze extra in half quart jars.

Recipe 618

CAJUN SEASONED RICE

The night before soak six cups of rice.

One tablespoon of BIOSALT

Eight cups of water into large pan.

The next day bring to a boil and then turn to low for 10 -15 minutes.

Place lid on, until rice is cooked.

Add the following:

Mix and place lid on pan and let sit for 15 minutes or more, (turn off heat first)

One tablespoon of paprika
One tablespoon of onion powder
One tablespoon of BIOSALT
Two tablespoons of cayenne
One tablespoon of garlic powder
One tablespoon of cumin

One teaspoon of MARJORAM

One teaspoon of thyme

Mix again

Serve hot -- can freeze extra in half quart jars.

Recipe 619

ORIENTAL SEASONED RICE

The night before soak six cups of rice.

One tablespoon of BIOSALT

Eight cups of water into large pan.

The next day bring to a boil and then turn to low for 10 -15 minutes.

Place lid on, until rice is cooked.

Add the following:

Mix and place lid on pan and let sit for 15 minutes or more, (turn off heat first)

-Two bell peppers cut small

(place in large pan while boiling rice)

One tablespoon of garlic powder
One tablespoon of onion powder
One tablespoon of BIOSALT
Two tablespoons of lemon rind

Two tablespoons of lemon powder

One half cup of sesame seeds

Mix

Serve hot -- can freeze extra in half quart jars.

Recipe 620

CAROB CASHEW CREAM PIE

Place the following into a vitamix:

One cup of Maple syrup

One cup of pineapple juice

One cup of water

One and one half cups of Cashews

One half cup of sucanant sugar

One cup of almond butter

One half cup of carob powder

Mix until smooth

For pie crust see special pie crust recipe number 38.

Pour the above into unbaked pie shell.

Bake 350 degrees 20 minutes

Let cool and serve cold -- refrigerate. Cut pie and can freeze extra.

Recipe 621

PERO CASHEW CREAM PIE

Place the following into a vitamix:

One cup of Maple syrup

One cup of pineapple juice

One cup of water

One and one half cups of Cashews

One half cup of sucanant sugar

One cup of almond butter

One half cup of Pero coffee

Mix until smooth

For pie crust see special pie crust recipe number 38.

Pour the above ingredients into unbaked pie shell.

Bake 350 degrees 20 minutes

Let cool and serve cold. Place in refrigerator.

Cut pie. Can freeze extra.

Recipe 622

CINNAMON CASHEW CREAM PIE

Place the following into a vitamix:

One cup of Maple syrup

One cup of pineapple juice

One cup of water

One and one half cups of Cashews

One half cup of sucanant sugar

One cup of almond butter

Two -- four tablespoons of cinnamon

This depends on how strong you want a cinnamon taste., always start with two tablespoons on first pie.

Blend until smooth

For pie crust see special pie crust recipe number 38.

Pour the above ingredients into unbaked pie shell.

Bake 350 degrees 20 minutes

Let cool and serve cold. Place in refrigerator.

Cut pie. Can freeze extra.

Recipe 623

LEMON CASHEW CREAM PIE

Place the following into a vitamix:

One cup of Maple syrup

One cup of pineapple juice

One cup of water

One and one half cups of Cashews

One half cup of sucanant sugar

One cup of almond butter

One fourth cup of whole wheat pastry flour

Two -- four tablespoons of Lemon Rind

This depends on how much lemon taste. you want, always start with two tablespoons
   on first pie.

Two tablespoons of lemon juice powder

Blend until smooth.

For pie crust see special pie crust recipe number 38.

Pour all above ingredients into unbaked pie shell.

Bake 350 degrees 20 minutes

Let cool and serve cold. Place in refrigerator.

Cut pie. Can freeze extra.

Recipe 624

ORANGE CASHEW CREAM PIE

Place the following into a vitamix:

One cup of Maple syrup

One cup of pineapple juice

One cup of water

One and one half cups of Cashews

One half cup of sucanant sugar

One cup of almond butter

One fourth cup of whole wheat pastry flour

Two tablespoons of lemon juice powder

Two -- four tablespoons of Orange Rind

This depends on how much orange taste. you want, always start with two tablespoons
on first pie.

Blend until smooth.

For pie crust see special pie crust recipe number 38.

Pour all above ingredients into unbaked pie shell.

Bake 350 degrees 20 minutes

Let cool and serve cold. Place in refrigerator.

Cut pie. Can freeze extra.

Recipe 625

SPICE CASHEW CREAM PIE

Place the following into a vitamix:

One cup of Maple syrup

One cup of pineapple juice

One cup of water

One and one half cups of Cashews

One half cup of sucanant sugar

One cup of almond butter

One fourth cup of whole wheat pastry flour

One half -- one teaspoon of clove powder

One half -- one teaspoon of cinnamon powder

One half -- one teaspoon of ginger powder

This depends on how much spice taste. you want, always start with a half teaspoon
  on first pie.

Blend all ingredients until smooth.

For pie crust see special pie crust recipe number 38.

Pour all above ingredients into unbaked pie shell.

Bake 350 degrees 20 minutes

Let cool and serve cold. Place in refrigerator.

Cut pie. Can freeze extra.

Recipe 626

LICORICE and CASHEW CREAM PIE

Place the following into a vitamix:

One cup of Maple syrup

One cup of pineapple juice

One cup of water

One and one half cups of Cashews

One half cup of sucanant sugar

One cup of almond butter

One fourth cup of whole wheat pastry flour

One fourth or one half teaspoon of liquid Anise

This depends on how much licorice taste. you want, always start with one fourth
teaspoon on first pie.

Blend all ingredients until smooth.

For pie crust see special pie crust recipe number 38.

Pour all above ingredients into unbaked pie shell.

Bake 350 degrees 20 minutes

Let cool and serve cold. Place in refrigerator.

Cut pie. Can freeze extra.

Recipe 627

GREEN HOT SAUCE

Place into a vitamix the following:

DO NOT ADD ANY WATER:

One onion

One -- two cups of green jalapeno peppers

Five cloves of garlic

Five tablespoons of Braggs

One tablespoon of cayenne pepper

One tablespoon of lemon rind

Two teaspoons of biosalt

One -- two cups of lime juice (fresh)

One cup of lemon juice

One fourth cup of maple syrup

Fifty tomatillos -- remove paper like skin and wash first. These tomatoes come in
    a variety of sizes.

Pour into a large pan and boil for two hours on low, let cool.

Place in half quart jars and freeze.

HELPFUL HINTS:

Since all tomatillos will not fit into vitamix at same time, you will need to blend
more than several containers full.

Recipe 628

GREEN SALSA

Place following in a vitamix:

DO NOT ADD ANY WATER

Fifty tomatillos -- these come in a variety of sizes -- remove paperlike skin and wash.

One tablespoon of cayenne pepper

Five tablespoons of Baggs

One tablespoon of lemon rind

two teaspoons of Biosalt

One -- two cups of lime juice (fresh)

One cup of lemon juice (fresh)

One fourth cup of maple syrup

Pour into a large pan and cut the following small and place into sauce pan:

One -- two cups of Green Jalapeno peppers

Five cloves of garlic

One onion

Boil for two hours on low and stir occasionally, let cool, can freeze in half quart jars.

HELPFUL HINTS:

All tomatillos will not fit into vitamix at same time, you will need to blend more than several container full.

Recipe 629

Sesame Seed Biscuits

Mix the following in a large bowl:

1 - 2 tablespoons of seasme seeds
2 cups of whole wheat pastry flour (sifted)
One half teaspoon of Biosalt
6 tablespoons of Almond Butter

Mix and set aside, until room temperature is achieved.

In a small cup place three fourths cup of finger warm soymilk and one tablespoon
of yeast or one packet.

One and one half teaspoon of Sucanant Sugar

Mix and pour into above bowl and mix again.

Let sit covered and place in a warm place for 10 - 20 minutes or more -- dough
should raise. Knead dough on a floured surface, with a rolling pin roll out dough
and use 2 x 2 inch cookie cutter to cut circles in dough.

Place on trays lined with cookie matt.

Bake 425 degrees 13 to 15 minutes

Helpful Hints:

This recipe makes 10 biscuits. Follow yeast instructions and cut circles one half inch thick. After biscuits cool, place in refrigerator and can consume 3 days after the harmful yeast gas is gone.

Recipe 630

Italian Biscuits

Mix the following in a large bowl:

1 - 2 teaspoons of Italian seasoning this depends on how strong you want your
   biscuits top taste Italian.
2 cups of whole wheat pastry flour (sifted)
One half teaspoon of Biosalt
6 tablespoons of Almond Butter

Mix and set aside, until room temperature is achieved.

In a small cup place three fourths cup of finger warm soymilk and one tablespoon
   of yeast or one packet.

One and one half teaspoon of Sucanant Sugar

Mix and pour into above bowl and mix again.

Let sit covered and place in a warm place for 10 - 20 minutes or more -- dough
   should raise. Knead dough on a floured surface, with a rolling pin roll out dough
   and use 2 x 2 inch cookie cutter to cut circles in dough.

Place on trays lined with cookie matt.

Bake 425 degrees 13 to 15 minutes

Helpful Hints:

This recipe makes 10 biscuits. Follow yeast instructions and cut circles one half inch thick. After biscuits cool, place in refrigerator and can consume 3 days after the harmful yeast gas is gone.

Recipe 631

Garlic Biscuits

Mix the following in a large bowl:

One half to one teaspoon of garlic powder this depends on how strong you want a garlic taste in yor biscuits.

2 cups of whole wheat pastry flour (sifted)

One half teaspoon of Biosalt

6 tablespoons of Almond Butter

Mix and set aside, until room temperature is achieved.

In a small cup place three fourths cup of finger warm soymilk and one tablespoon of yeast or one packet.

One and one half teaspoon of Sucanant Sugar

Mix and pour into above bowl and mix again.

Let sit covered and place in a warm place for 10 - 20 minutes or more -- dough should raise. Knead dough on a floured surface, with a rolling pin roll out dough and use 2 x 2 inch cookie cutter to cut circles in dough.

Place on trays lined with cookie matt.

Bake 425 degrees 13 to 15 minutes

Helpful Hints:

This recipe makes 10 biscuits. Follow yeast instructions and cut circles one half inch thick. After biscuits cool, place in refrigerator and can consume 3 days after the harmful yeast gas is gone.

Recipe 632

Hot Biscuits

Mix the following in a large bowl:

One half to one teaspoon of Cayane pepper, this depends on how hot you desire
   your biscuits to be.

2 cups of whole wheat pastry flour (sifted)

One half teaspoon of Biosalt

6 tablespoons of Almond Butter

Mix and set aside, until room temperature is achieved.

In a small cup place three fourths cup of finger warm soymilk and one tablespoon
   of yeast or one packet.

One and one half teaspoon of Sucanant Sugar

Mix and pour into above bowl and mix again.

Let sit covered and place in a warm place for 10 - 20 minutes or more -- dough
   should raise. Knead dough on a floured surface, with a rolling pin roll out dough
   and use 2 x 2 inch cookie cutter to cut circles in dough.

Place on trays lined with cookie matt.

Bake 425 degrees 13 to 15 minutes

Helpful Hints:

This recipe makes 10 biscuits. Follow yeast instructions and cut circles one half inch thick. After biscuits cool, place in refrigerator and can consume 3 days after the harmful yeast gas is gone.

Recipe 633

Soymilk Biscuits

Mix the following in a large bowl:

2 cups of whole wheat pastry flour (sifted)

One half teaspoon of Biosalt

6 tablespoons of Almond Butter

Mix and set aside, until room temperature is achieved.

In a small cup place three fourths cup of finger warm soymilk and one tablespoon of yeast or one packet.

One and one half teaspoon of Sucanant Sugar

Mix and pour into above bowl and mix again.

Let sit covered and place in a warm place for 10 - 20 minutes or more -- dough should raise. Knead dough on a floured surface, with a rolling pin roll out dough and use 2 x 2 inch cookie cutter to cut circles in dough.

Place on trays lined with cookie matt.

Bake 425 degrees 13 to 15 minutes

Helpful Hints:

This recipe makes 10 biscuits. Follow yeast instructions and cut circles one half inch thick. After biscuits cool, place in refrigerator and can consume 3 days after the harmful yeast gas is gone.

Recipe 634

Poppy Seed Biscuits

Mix the following in a large bowl:

1 - 2 tablespoons of poppy seeds
2 cups of whole wheat pastry flour (sifted)
One half teaspoon of Biosalt
6 tablespoons of Almond Butter

Mix and set aside, until room temperature is achieved.

In a small cup place three fourths cup of finger warm soymilk and one tablespoon
of yeast or one packet.

One and one half teaspoon of Sucanant Sugar

Mix and pour into above bowl and mix again.

Let sit covered and place in a warm place for 10 - 20 minutes or more -- dough
should raise. Knead dough on a floured surface, with a rolling pin roll out dough
and use 2 x 2 inch cookie cutter to cut circles in dough.

Place on trays lined with cookie matt.

Bake 425 degrees 13 to 15 minutes

Helpful Hints:

This recipe makes 10 biscuits. Follow yeast instructions and cut circles one half inch thick. After biscuits cool, place in refrigerator and can consume 3 days after the harmful yeast gas is gone.

Recipe 635

GUSTAVO RIOS SR. LEMON PIE COOKIES

Mix in a large bowl the following:

2 cups of sucanant sugar

one fourth cup of tofu

1 cup of almond butter

one half cup of lemon rind

Mix and add 2 cups of whole wheat pastry flour (sifted)

Mix again and place into a 9 x 9 inch cake pan, lined with parchment paper.

Press into pan with backside of a spoon.

Add one cup of chopped walnuts on top of pan; and press into dough.

Bake 275 degrees one hour

Recipe 636

HORTINCIA RIOS SPICE PIE COOKIES

Mix in a large bowl the following:

2 cups of sucanant sugar

one fourth cup of tofu

1 cup of almond butter

1 teaspoon of clove powder

1 teaspoon of cinnamon

1 teaspoon of ginger

Mix and add 2 cups of whole wheat pastry flour (sifted)

Mix again and place into a 9 x 9 inch cake pan, lined with parchment paper.

Press into pan with backside of a spoon.

Add one cup of chopped walnuts on top of pan; and press into dough.

Bake 275 degrees one hour

Let cool and cut into pie shapes.

This recipe makes 16 parts.

Recipe 637

ORANGE PIE COOKIES

Mix in a large bowl the following:

2 cups of sucanant sugar

one fourth cup of tofu

1 cup of almond butter

one half cup of orange rind

Mix and add 2 cups of whole wheat pastry flour (sifted)

Mix again and place into a 9 x 9 inch cake pan,

lined with parchment paper.

Press into pan with backside of a spoon.

Add one cup of chopped walnuts on top of pan; and press into dough.

Bake 275 degrees one hour

Let cool and cut into pie shapes.

This recipe makes 16 parts.

DATE PIE COOKIES

Mix in a large bowl the following:

2 cups of sucanant sugar

one fourth cup of tofu

1 cup of almond butter

Mix and add 2 cups of whole wheat pastry flour (sifted)

Mix again and place into a 9 x 9 inch cake pan,

lined with parchment paper.

Press into pan with backside of a spoon.

Add one and one half cups of chopped dates on top of pan; and press into dough.

Bake 275 degrees one hour

Let cool and cut into pie shapes.

This recipe makes 16 parts.

Recipe 639

CASHEW AND CAROB ICE CREAM

Place into vitamix the following:

One fourth teaspoon of Biosalt

2 cups of Cashews

2 cups of walnuts

3 cups of Puffed Rice

2 cups of maple syrup

1 tablespoon of almond butter

One half cup of carob powder

3 cups of water

Blend until smooth.

Place in one half pint jars and freeze.

CASHEW, CAROB, COFFEE ICE CREAM

Place in a vitamix the following:

2 cups of cashews

2 cups of walnuts

3 cups of puffed rice

one fourth teaspoon of biosalt

2 tablespoons of Pero coffee powder

2 cups of maple syrup

one half cup of carob powder

3 cups of water

Blend until smooth.

Place into one half pint jars and freeze.

Recipe 641

CASHEW PUMPKIN ICE CREAM

Place in a vitamix the following:

One fourth teaspoon of biosalt

2 cups of cashews

2 cups of walnuts

3 cups of puffed rice

2 cups of maple syrup

1 tablespoon of almond butter

3 cups of water

Blend until smooth.

Place into one half pint jars and freeze.

Recipe 642

CASHEW ORANGE ICE CREAM

Place in a vitamix the following:

One fourth teaspoon of biosalt

2 cups of cashews

2 cups of walnuts

3 cups of puffed rice

2 cups of maple syrup

1 tablespoon of almond butter

3 cups of water

Blend until smooth.

Place into one half pint jars and freeze.

Recipe 643

CASHEW PINEAPPLE ICE CREAM

Place in a vitamix the following:

One fourth teaspoon of biosalt

2 cups of cashews

2 cups of walnuts

3 cups of puffed rice

1 cup of pineapple juice

2 cups of maple syrup

1 tablespoon of almond butter

3 cups of water

Blend until smooth.

Place into one half pint jars and freeze.

Recipe 644

CASHEW RAISIN ICE CREAM

Place in a vitamix the following:

One fourth teaspoon of biosalt

2 cups of cashews

2 cups of walnuts

3 cups of puffed rice

2 cups of claned raisins

wash and let drain for 1 hour

2 cups of maple syrup

1 tablespoon of almond butter

3 cups of water

Blend until smooth.

Place into one half pint jars and freeze.

Recipe 645

CASHEW APRICOT ICE CREAM

Place in a vitamix the following:

One fourth teaspoon of biosalt

2 cups of cashews

2 cups of walnuts

3 cups of puffed rice

2 cups of maple syrup

1 tablespoon of almond butter

3 cups of water

1 cup of apricots (remove seeds only)

Blend until smooth.

Place into one half pint jars and freeze.

Recipe 646

CASHEW LICORICE ICE CREAM

Place in a vitamix the following:

One fourth teaspoon of biosalt

2 cups of cashews

2 cups of walnuts

3 cups of puffed rice

one fourth to one half teaspoon of anise- this depends on how strong you desire a
    licorice taste- start first recipe with one fourth teaspoon

2 cups of maple syrup

1 tablespoon of almond butter

3 cups of water

Blend until smooth.

Place into one half pint jars and freeze.

Recipe 647

CASHEW SPICE ICE CREAM

Place in a vitamix the following:

One fourth teaspoon of biosalt

2 cups of cashews

2 cups of walnuts

3 cups of puffed rice

2 cups of maple syrup

1 tablespoon of almond butter

one half to one teaspoon of cinnamon

one fourth to one half teaspoon of clove powder

one half to one teaspoon of ginger this depends on how strong of spice taste you
desire, always start first recipe with lesser amount of spice.

3 cups of water

Blend until smooth.

Place into one half pint jars and freeze.

CASHEW COFFEE ICE CREAM

Place in a vitamix the following:

One fourth teaspoon of biosalt

2 cups of cashews

2 cups of walnuts

3 cups of puffed rice

one half cup of Pero

2 cups of maple syrup

1 tablespoon of almond butter

one half cup of carob powder

3 cups of water

Blend until smooth.

Place into one half pint jars and freeze.

Recipe 649

CASHEW LEMON ICE CREAM

Place in a vitamix the following:

One fourth teaspoon of biosalt

2 cups of cashews

2 cups of walnuts

3 cups of puffed rice

1 cup of lemon rind

2 cups of maple syrup

1 tablespoon of almond butter

one half cup of carob powder

3 cups of water

Blend until smooth.

Place into one half pint jars and freeze.

Recipe 650

CASHEW CINNAMON ICE CREAM

Place in a vitamix the following:

One fourth teaspoon of biosalt

2 cups of cashews

2 cups of walnuts

3 cups of puffed rice

1 to 2 tablespoons of cinnamon- this depends on how much cinnamon tast you
    desire-always start with one tablespoon on first recipe.

2 cups of maple syrup

1 tablespoon of almond butter

3 cups of water

Blend until smooth.

Place into one half pint jars and freeze.

Recipe 651

CASHEW PEPPERMINT ICE CREAM

Place in a vitamix the following:

One fourth teaspoon of biosalt

2 cups of cashews

2 cups of walnuts

3 cups of puffed rice

2 cups of maple syrup

1 tablespoon of almond butter

3 cups of water

one fourth to one half teaspoon of liquid peppermint - this depends on how strong
   a peppermint taste you desire- always start first recipe with one fourth teaspoon.

Blend until smooth.

Place into one half pint jars and freeze.

Recipe 652

CASHEW PERO PEPPERMINT ICE CREAM

Place in a vitamix the following:

One fourth teaspoon of biosalt

2 cups of cashews

2 cups of walnuts

3 cups of puffed rice

2 cups of maple syrup

1 tablespoon of almond butter

3 cups of water

2 tablespoons of Pero coffee powder

one fourth to one half teaspoon of liquid peppermint- this depends on how strong a peppermint taste you desire - always start with first recipe with one fourth teaspoon.

Blend until smooth.

Place into one half pint jars and freeze.

Recipe 653

CASHEW BLUEBERRY ICE CREAM

Place in a vitamix the following:

One fourth teaspoon of biosalt

2 cups of cashews

2 cups of walnuts

3 cups of puffed rice

2 cups of maple syrup

1 tablespoon of almond butter

3 cups of water

1 cup of blueberries

Blend until smooth.

Place into one half pint jars and freeze.

Recipe 654

CASHEW CHERRY ICE CREAM

Place in a vitamix the following:

One fourth teaspoon of biosalt

2 cups of cashews

2 cups of walnuts

3 cups of puffed rice

2 cups of maple syrup

1 tablespoon of almond butter

3 cups of water

1 cup of cherries

(remove stems and seeds)

Blend until smooth.

Place into one half pint jars and freeze.

Recipe 655

CASHEW NECTARINE ICE CREAM

Place in a vitamix the following:

One fourth teaspoon of biosalt

2 cups of cashews

2 cups of walnuts

3 cups of puffed rice

2 cups of maple syrup

1 tablespoon of almond butter

3 cups of water

1 cup of nectarines

(remove pits and stems)

Blend until smooth.

Place into one half pint jars and freeze.

Recipe 656

CASHEW STRAWBERRY ICE CREAM

Place in a vitamix the following:

One fourth teaspoon of biosalt

2 cups of cashews

2 cups of walnuts

3 cups of puffed rice

2 cups of maple syrup

1 tablespoon of almond butter

3 cups of water

2 cups of strawberries

Blend until smooth.

Place into one half pint jars and freeze.

Recipe 657

CASHEW PEACH ICE CREAM

Place in a vitamix the following:

One fourth teaspoon of biosalt

2 cups of cashews

2 cups of walnuts

3 cups of puffed rice

2 cups of maple syrup

1 tablespoon of almond butter

3 cups of water

1 cup of peaches

(minus pits and stems)

Blend until smooth.

Place into one half pint jars and freeze.

Recipe 658

CASHEW ORANGE PINEAPPLE ICE CREAM

Place in a vitamix the following:

One fourth teaspoon of biosalt

2 cups of cashews

2 cups of walnuts

3 cups of puffed rice

2 cups of maple syrup

1 tablespoon of almond butter

3 cups of water

1 cup of pineapple juice

3 to 6 tablespoons orange rind

Blend until smooth.

Place into one half pint jars and freeze.

Recipe 659

CASHEW LEMON PINEAPPLE ICE CREAM

Place in a vitamix the following:

One fourth teaspoon of biosalt

2 cups of cashews

2 cups of walnuts

3 cups of puffed rice

2 cups of maple syrup

1 tablespoon of almond butter

3 cups of water

1 cup of pineapple juice

3 - 6 tablespoons of lemon rind

Blend until smooth.

Place into one half pint jars and freeze.

Recipe 660

LEMON SUCANANT SUGAR COOKIES

Place the following into a vitamix and blend until smooth:

2 teaspoon of pineapple juice or water.

3 cups of maple syrup

3 -- 5 tablespoons of lemon rind this depends on how much lemon taste you desire
   -- on first recipe use 3 tablespoons.

3 cups of almond butter

1 teaspoon of vanilla

Mix and pour into large bowl and add:

4 cups of whole wheat pastry flour (sifted)

Mix dough the day before -- place in refrigerator covered

The next day roll out dough instead of using flour on board -- pour sucanant sugar.

Using a rolling pin make dough cookie thickness.

Can use any cookie cutter or shape.

Best to use a 3 x 3 inch circle.

For this recipe 1 -- 2 pounds of sucanant sugar is required.

Place on trays lined with cookie mat 9 per tray.

Bake 10 -- 13 minutes 375 degrees

Recipe 661

ORANGE SUCANANT SUGAR COOKIES

Place the following into a vitamix and blend until smooth:

2 teaspoon of pineapple juice or water.

3 cups of maple syrup

3 -- 5 tablespoons of orange rind this depends on how much orange taste you desire
-- on first recipe use 3 tablespoons.

3 cups of almond butter

1 teaspoon of vanilla

Mix and pour into large bowl and add:

4 cups of whole wheat pastry flour (sifted)

Mix dough the day before -- place in refrigerator covered

The next day roll out dough instead of using flour on board -- pour sucanant sugar.

Using a rolling pin make dough cookie thickness.

Can use any cookie cutter or shape.

Best to use a 3 x 3 inch circle.

For this recipe 1 -- 2 pounds of sucanant sugar is required.

Place on trays lined with cookie mat 9 per tray.

Bake 10 -- 13 minutes 375 degrees

Recipe 662

COCONUT CASHEW CREAM PIE

Place following into a vitamix.

Blend until smooth,

1 cup of maple syrup

one fourth teaspoon of biosalt

2 cups of coconut lite

one half cup of sucanant sugar

one fourth cup of whole wheat pastry flour

1 cup of almond butter

1 cup of water

1 cup of pineapple juice

1 and a half cups of cashews

Mix until smooth.

Pour into unbaked pie shell,

(see recipe # 38)

Bake 350 degrees 20 minutes

Let cool. Place in refrigerator.

Serve cold.

PLUM FRUIT ROLL

The day before wash 6 pounds of plums -- let dry and place in refrigerator.

The next day remove leaves, stems and seeds.

Then place into vitamix with 4 tablespoons of orange rind.

Blend until smooth. Do not add any water.

Pour into a large tall pan.

Boil on low for 30 minutes.

Helpful Hints: If oven has 2 grills remove, place 2 cookie mats on each grill.

Overlap to fit.

(four mats needed) If oven has one grill cut recipe into one half.

Pour mixture from pan and spread thin on mats. Place grills back into oven

(in center of oven) then turn heat to the lowest warm.

Bake 15 - 20 hours.

This is a long process - however fruit must be dried and a thin leather texture appearance.

I recommend place in oven overnight when oven is not being used.

The next day fruit will be dried

Let cool and store in refrigerator. Sometimes depending on how thick fruit is on mat, fruit may take longer to dry.

CHERRY FRUIT ROLL

The day before wash 6 pounds of cherries--let dry and then place in refrigerator.

The next day remove stems, leaves and seeds.

Then place into vitamix.

Blend until smooth. Do not add any water.

Pour into a large tall pan. Boil on low for 30 minutes.

Helpful Hints: If oven has 2 grills remove, place 2 cookie mats on each grill.

Overlap to fit. (four mats needed)

If oven has one grill cut recipe into one half.

Pour mixture from pan and spread thin on mats.

Place grills back into oven (in center of oven) then turn heat to the lowest warm.

Bake 15 - 20 hours. This is a long process - however fruit must be dried and a thin leather texture appearance.

I recommend place in oven overnight when oven is not being used.

The next day fruit will be dried.

Let cool and store in refrigerator. Sometimes depending on how thick fruit is on
mat, fruit may take longer to dry.

LICORICE PLUM FRUIT ROLL

The day before wash 6 pounds of plums -- let dry and then place in refrigerator.

The next day remove stems, leaves and seeds.

Then place into vitamix. Blend until smooth.

Do not add any water.

Pour into a large tall pan. Boil on low for 30 minutes, and add 1 - 2 teaspoons of anise.

Stir occasionally.

Helpful Hints: If oven has 2 grills remove, place 2 cookie mats on each grill.

Overlap to fit. (four mats needed)

If oven has one grill cut recipe into one half.

Pour mixture from pan and spread thin on mats.

Place grills back into oven (in center of oven) then turn heat to the lowest warm.

Bake 15 - 20 hours. This is a long process - however fruit must be dried and a thin leather texture appearance.

I recommend place in oven overnight when oven is not being used.

The next day fruit will be dried.

Let cool and store in refrigerator. Sometimes depending on how thick fruit is on mat, fruit may take longer to dry.

Recipe 666

DATE & PLUM ICE CREAM

Place into vitamix the following:

One fourth teaspoon of Biosalt

One half cup of soy milk

2 cups of walnuts

1 pound or 1 brick of Tofu

3 cups of Puffed Corn or Rice

1 tablespoon of Almond butter

2 pitted plums

½ c pitted dates

2 cups of maple syrup

Blend until smooth

Pour into 6 ounce glass jars and freeze

Recipe 667

GRAPEFRUIT ICE CREAM

Place into vitamix the following:

One fourth teaspoon of Biosalt

One half cup of soy milk

2 cups of walnuts

1 pound or 1 brick of Tofu

3 cups of Puffed Corn or Rice

1 tablespoon of Almond butter

3 - 6 tablespoons of Grapefruit juice

2 cups of maple syrup

Blend until smooth

Pour into 6 ounce glass jars and freeze

Recipe 668

PEACH FRUIT ROLL

The day before wash 6 pounds of peaches -- let dry and place in refrigerator.

The next day remove leaves, stems, and seeds.

Then place into vitamix. Blend until smooth.

Do not add any water.

Pour into a large tall pan. Boil on low for 30 minutes.

Helpful Hints: If oven has 2 grills remove, place 2 cookie mats on each grill.

Overlap to fit. (four mats needed) If oven has one grill cut recipe into one half.

Pour mixture from pan and spread thin on mats.

Place grills back into oven (in center of oven) then turn heat to the lowest warm.

Bake 15 - 20 hours.

This is a long process - however fruit must be dried and a thin leather texture appearance.

I recommend place in oven overnight when oven is not being used.

The next day fruit will be dried.

Let cool and store in refrigerator. Sometimes depending on how thick fruit is on mat, fruit may take longer to dry.

APRICOT FRUIT ROLL

The day before wash 6 pounds of apricots-- let dry and place in refrigerator.

The next day remove leaves, stems, and seeds.

Then place into vitamix. Blend until smooth. Do not add any water.

Pour into a large tall pan. Boil on low for 30 minutes.

Helpful Hints: If oven has 2 grills remove, place 2 cookie mats on each grill.

Overlap to fit. (four mats needed) If oven has one grill cut recipe into one half.

Pour mixture from pan and spread thin on mats. Place grills back into oven (in center of oven) then turn heat to the lowest warm.

Bake 15 - 20 hours. This is a long process - however fruit must be dried and a thin leather texture appearance.

I recommend place in oven overnight when oven is not being used.

The next day fruit will be dried. Let cool and store in refrigerator. Sometimes depending on how thick fruit is on mat, fruit may take longer to dry.

Recipe 670

STRAWBERRY FRUIT ROLL

The day before wash 6 pounds of strawberries -- let dry and place in refrigerator.

The next day remove cores.

Then place into vitamix. Blend until smooth.

Do not add any water.

Pour into a large tall pan. Boil on low for 30 minutes.

Helpful Hints: If oven has 2 grills remove, place 2 cookie mats on each grill.

Overlap to fit. (four mats needed) If oven has one grill cut recipe into one half.

Pour mixture from pan and spread thin on mats. Place grills back into oven (in center of oven) then turn heat to the lowest warm.

Bake 15 - 20 hours. This is a long process - however fruit must be dried and a thin leather texture appearance.

I recommend place in oven overnight when oven is not being used.

The next day fruit will be dried. Let cool and store in refrigerator. Sometimes depending on how thick fruit is on mat, fruit may take longer to dry.

PEAR FRUIT ROLL

The day before wash 6 pounds of pears -- let dry and place in refrigerator.

The next day remove cores.

Then place into vitamix. Blend until smooth.

Do not add any water.

Pour into a large tall pan. Boil on low for 30 minutes.

Helpful Hints: If oven has 2 grills remove, place 2 cookie mats on each grill.

Overlap to fit. (four mats needed) If oven has one grill cut recipe into one half.

Pour mixture from pan and spread thin on mats. Place grills back into oven (in center of oven) then turn heat to the lowest warm.

Bake 15 - 20 hours. This is a long process - however fruit must be dried and a thin leather texture appearance.

I recommend place in oven overnight when oven is not being used.

The next day fruit will be dried. Let cool and store in refrigerator. Sometimes depending on how thick fruit is on mat, fruit may take longer to dry.

Recipe 672

NECTARINE FRUIT ROLL

The day before wash 6 pounds of Nectarines-- let dry and place in refrigerator.

The next day remove stems, leaves and seeds.

Then place into vitamix. Blend until smooth. Do not add any water.

Pour into a large tall pan. Boil on low for 30 minutes.

Helpful Hints: If oven has 2 grills remove, place 2 cookie mats on each grill.

Overlap to fit. (four mats needed) If oven has one grill cut recipe into one half.

Pour mixture from pan and spread thin on mats. Place grills back into oven (in center of oven) then turn heat to the lowest warm.

Bake 15 - 20 hours. This is a long process - however fruit must be dried and a thin leather texture appearance.

I recommend place in oven overnight when oven is not being used.

The next day fruit will be dried. Let cool and store in refrigerator. Sometimes depending on how thick fruit is on mat, fruit may take longer to dry.

Recipe 673

BLACKBERRY FRUIT ROLL

The day before wash 6 pounds of blackberries -- let dry and place in refrigerator.

The next day remove stems.

Then place into vitamix. Blend until smooth. Do not add any water.

Pour into a large tall pan. Boil on low for 30 minutes.

Helpful Hints: If oven has 2 grills remove, place 2 cookie mats on each grill.

Overlap to fit. (four mats needed) If oven has one grill cut recipe into one half.

Pour mixture from pan and spread thin on mats. Place grills back into oven (in center of oven) then turn heat to the lowest warm.

Bake 15 - 20 hours.

This is a long process - however fruit must be dried and a thin leather texture appearance.

I recommend place in oven overnight when oven is not being used.

The next day fruit will be dried. Let cool and store in refrigerator. Sometimes depending on how thick fruit is on mat, fruit may take longer to dry.

Recipe 674

PINEAPPLE FRUIT ROLL

Drain the juice from 6 pounds of pineapple (can) or can use fresh pineapple.

Then place into vitamix. Blend until smooth. Do not add any water.

Pour into a large tall pan. Boil on low for 30 minutes.

Helpful Hints: If oven has 2 grills remove, place 2 cookie mats on each grill.

Overlap to fit. (four mats needed) If oven has one grill cut recipe into one half.

Pour mixture from pan and spread thin on mats. Place grills back into oven (in center of oven) then turn heat to the lowest warm.

Bake 15 - 20 hours. This is a long process - however fruit must be dried and a thin leather texture appearance.

I recommend place in oven overnight when oven is not being used.

The next day fruit will be dried. Let cool and store in refrigerator.

Sometimes depending on how thick fruit is on mat, fruit may take longer to dry.

Recipe 675

APPLE FRUIT ROLL

The day before wash 6 pounds of apple -- let dry and place in refrigerator.

The next day remove core only.

Then place into vitamix. Blend until smooth.

Do not add any water.

Pour into a large tall pan. Boil on low for 30 minutes.

Helpful Hints: If oven has 2 grills remove, place 2 cookie mats on each grill.

Overlap to fit. (four mats needed) If oven has one grill cut recipe into one half.

Pour mixture from pan and spread thin on mats. Place grills back into oven (in center of oven) then turn heat to the lowest warm.

Bake 15 - 20 hours. This is a long process - however fruit must be dried and a thin leather texture appearance.

I recommend place in oven overnight when oven is not being used.

The next day fruit will be dried. Let cool and store in refrigerator. Sometimes depending on how thick fruit is on mat, fruit may take longer to dry.

Recipe 676

ORANGE PLUM FRUIT ROLL

The day before wash 6 pounds of plums -- let dry and place in refrigerator.

The next day remove leaves, stems and seeds.

Then place into vitamix with 4 tablespoons of orange rind. Blend until smooth. Do not add any water.

Pour into a large tall pan. Boil on low for 30 minutes.

Helpful Hints: If oven has 2 grills remove, place 2 cookie mats on each grill.

Overlap to fit. (four mats needed) If oven has one grill cut recipe into one half.

Pour mixture from pan and spread thin on mats. Place grills back into oven (in center of oven) then turn heat to the lowest warm.

Bake 15 - 20 hours. This is a long process - however fruit must be dried and a thin leather texture appearance.

I recommend place in oven overnight when oven is not being used.

The next day fruit will be dried. Let cool and store in refrigerator. Sometimes depending on how thick fruit is on mat, fruit may take longer to dry.

LEMON PLUM FRUIT ROLL

The day before wash 6 pounds of plums -- let dry and place in refrigerator.

The next day remove leaves, stems, and seeds.

Then place into vitamix with 4 tablespoons of lemon rind. Blend until smooth. Do not add any water.

Pour into a large tall pan. Boil on low for 30 minutes.

Helpful Hints: If oven has 2 grills remove, place 2 cookie mats on each grill.

Overlap to fit. (four mats needed) If oven has one grill cut recipe into one half.

Pour mixture from pan and spread thin on mats. Place grills back into oven (in center of oven) then turn heat to the lowest warm.

Bake 15 - 20 hours. This is a long process - however fruit must be dried and a thin leather texture appearance.

I recommend place in oven overnight when oven is not being used.

The next day fruit will be dried. Let cool and store in refrigerator. Sometimes depending on how thick fruit is on mat, fruit may take longer to dry.

Recipe 678

GRAPEFRUIT PLUM FRUIT ROLL

The day before wash 6 pounds of plums -- let dry and place in refrigerator.

The next day remove leaves, stems and seeds.

Then place into vitamix with 6 tablespoons of grapefruit rind. Blend until smooth. Do not add any water.

Pour into a large tall pan. Boil on low for 30 minutes.

Helpful Hints: If oven has 2 grills remove, place 2 cookie mats on each grill.

Overlap to fit. (four mats needed) If oven has one grill cut recipe into one half.

Pour mixture from pan and spread thin on mats. Place grills back into oven (in center of oven) then turn heat to the lowest warm.

Bake 15 - 20 hours. This is a long process - however fruit must be dried and a thin leather texture appearance.

I recommend place in oven overnight when oven is not being used.

The next day fruit will be dried. Let cool and store in refrigerator. Sometimes depending on how thick fruit is on mat, fruit may take longer to dry.

PEPPERMINT PLUM FRUIT ROLL

The day before wash 6 pounds of plums -- let dry and return to the refrigerator.

The next day remove leaves, stems, and seeds.

Then place into vitamix with one fourth or one half teaspoon of peppermint liquid. This depends on how strong you want a peppermint taste, on first recipe use one fourth teaspoon.

Blend until smooth. Do not add any water.

Pour into a large tall pan. Boil on low for 30 minutes.

Helpful Hints: If oven has 2 grills remove, place 2 cookie mats on each grill.

Overlap to fit. (four mats needed) If oven has one grill cut recipe into one half.

Pour mixture from pan and spread thin on mats. Place grills back into oven (in center of oven) then turn heat to the lowest warm.

Bake 15 - 20 hours. This is a long process - however fruit must be dried and a thin leather texture appearance.

I recommend place in oven overnight when oven is not being used.

The next day fruit will be dried. Let cool and store in refrigerator. Sometimes depending on how thick fruit is on mat, fruit may take longer to dry.

Recipe 680

MARK D DAWSON ASIAN HOT SAUCE

Place the following into vitamix until smooth: making several batches adding

5 lbs red chile peppers

2c maple syrup

2 tablespoon garlic powder

2 tablespoon biosalt

2c lemon juice

20-25c water

Pour into a large pan boil for 2 hours on low and stir occasionally

store into 12 ounce jars and freeze

-

Recipe 681

GREEN ASIAN HOT SAUCE

Place in a vitamixes the following and blend until smooth.

5 pounds of green chili peppers (cleaned)

2 cups of maple syrup

2 tablespoons of garlic powder

2 tablespoons of biosalt

2 cups of lemon juice

20 -- 25 cups of water -- this depends on how thick or thin you want your sauce.

Place into large pan -- boil for 2 hours on low.

Let cool and pour into 6 ounce jars and freeze.

VANILLA PLUM FRUIT ROLL

The day before wash 6 pounds of plums -- let dry and then place in refrigerator.

The next day remove stems, leaves and seeds.

Then place into vitamix with 3 tablespoons of vanilla. Blend until smooth. Do not add any water.

Pour into a large tall pan. Boil on low for 30 minutes.

Helpful Hints: If oven has 2 grills remove, place 2 cookie mats on each grill.

Overlap to fit. (four mats needed) If oven has one grill cut recipe into one half.

Pour mixture from pan and spread thin on mats. Place grills back into oven (in center of oven) then turn heat to the lowest warm.

Bake 15 - 20 hours. This is a long process - however fruit must be dried and a thin leather texture appearance.

I recommend place in oven overnight when oven is not being used.

The next day fruit will be dried. Let cool and store in refrigerator. Sometimes depending on how thick fruit is on mat, fruit may take longer to dry.

Recipe 683

CASHEW COCONUT ICE CREAM

Place in a vitamix the following:

The juice of a fresh coconut

1 cup of fresh coconut

3 cups of water

2 cups of walnuts

3 cups of puffed rice

2 cups of cashews

2 cups of maple syrup

1 tablespoon of almond butter

one fourth teaspoon of biosalt

Blend until smooth and pour into

one half pint jars and freeze.

Recipe 684

COCONUT ICE CREAM

Place in a vitamix the following:

The juice of a fresh coconut

1 cup of fresh coconut

3 cups of water

2 cups of walnuts

3 cups of puffed rice

2 cups of maple syrup

1 tablespoon of almond butter

one fourth teaspoon of biosalt

Blend until smooth and pour into

one half pint jars and freeze.

Recipe 685

CANTALOUPE FRUIT ROLL

The day before wash cantaloupes and let dry and place in refrigerator.

The next day place 6 pounds of cantaloupes in vitamix minus seeds and skins.

Blend until smooth. Do not add any water.

Pour into a large tall pan. Boil on low for 30 minutes.

Helpful Hints: If oven has 2 grills remove, place 2 cookie mats on each grill.

Overlap to fit. (four mats needed) If oven has one grill cut recipe into one half.

Pour mixture from pan and spread thin on mats. Place grills back into oven (in center of oven) then turn heat to the lowest warm.

Bake 15 - 20 hours. This is a long process - however fruit must be dried and a thin leather texture appearance.

I recommend place in oven overnight when oven is not being used.

The next day fruit will be dried. Let cool and store in refrigerator. Sometimes depending on how thick fruit is on mat, fruit may take longer to dry.

MANGO FRUIT ROLL

The day before wash mangos--let dry and then place in refrigerator.

The next day remove skin and seeds.

Then place into vitamix the total of 6 pounds. Blend until smooth.

Do not add any water.

Pour into a large tall pan. Boil on low for 30 minutes.

Helpful Hints: If oven has 2 grills remove, place 2 cookie mats on each grill.

Overlap to fit. (total of four mats needed)

If oven has one grill cut recipe into one half.

Pour mixture from pan and spread thin on mats.

Place grills back into oven (in center of oven) then turn heat to the lowest warm.

Bake 15 - 20 hours. This is a long process - however fruit must be dried and a thin
leather texture appearance.

I recommend place in oven overnight when oven is not being used.

The next day fruit will be dried.

Let cool and store in refrigerator. Sometimes depending on how thick fruit is on
mat, fruit may take longer to dry.

PAPAYA FRUIT ROLL

The day before wash papaya -- let dry and place in refrigerator.

The next day remove skin and seeds.

Then place into vitamix 6 pounds of papaya. Blend until smooth. Do not add any water.

Pour into a large tall pan. Boil on low for 30 minutes.

Helpful Hints: If oven has 2 grills remove, place 2 cookie mats on each grill.

Overlap to fit. (four mats needed) If oven has one grill cut recipe into one half.

Pour mixture from pan and spread thin on mats. Place grills back into oven (in center of oven) then turn heat to the lowest warm.

Bake 15 - 20 hours. This is a long process - however fruit must be dried and a thin leather texture appearance.

I recommend place in oven overnight when oven is not being used.

The next day fruit will be dried. Let cool and store in refrigerator. Sometimes depending on how thick fruit is on mat, fruit may take longer to dry.

Recipe 688

GREEN HABANERO PEPPER HOT SAUCE

Place following in a vitamix:

2 and a half pounds of habaneros

2 and a half pounds of green peppers

(remove stems)

2 cups of maple syrup

2 cups of lemon juice

2 tablespoons of biosalt

20 -- 25 cups of water this depends on how thick or thin you want your sauce.

Boil on low for 2 hours.

Stir occasionally. Let cool, pour into 6 ounce jars.

Can freeze extra.

Recipe 689

HABANERO AND RED PEPPER HOT SAUCE

Place following in a vitamix:

2 and a half pounds of habaneros

2 and a half pounds of red peppers

(remove stems)

2 cups of maple syrup

2 cups of lemon juice

2 tablespoons of biosalt

20 -- 25 cups of water this depends on how thick or thin you want your sauce.

Boil on low for 2 hours.

Stir occasionally. Let cool, pour into 6 ounce jars.

Can freeze extra.

Recipe 690

CELERY AND HAVENERO RICE

The night before place 6 cups of rice and 8 cups of water into a large pan and set aside.

The next day add to the large pan the following:

8 - 12 habanero peppers cut small

6 stalks of celery cut small

1 tablespoon of biosalt

6 tablespoons of braggs

2 tablespoons of almond butter

Bring to a boil then turn to low for approximately 10 - 15 minutes, or until cooked.

Stir occasionally. Place lid on pan.

Serve hot. Can freeze extra in one half pint jars.

Recipe 691

LEMON -ORANGE-LIME GRAPEFRUIT POWDER

Wash and clean any of the above and let dry.

Cut three - eighths of an inch (the thickness approximately) remove seeds and stems,

Remove oven grills - if oven has 2 grills - use both. If oven has only one proceed.

Place 2 cookie mats on grills overlap, place slices on top - do not overlap.

Turn oven to warm for 15 - 20 hours, If slices are too thick - this will take longer
  to dry. Slices will be dry - Let cool and place several into

vitamix. Make into a fine powder.

Can store in glass jars one pint and freeze. This is a long process, however this will
  save time and money and has many uses, cakes, pies, ice cream, cookies, candy,
  and even sauces.

Recipe 692

SPICY CATSUP

Place the following in a vitamix.

Blend until smooth.

1 and a half cups of tomato paste

1 and a half cups of water

1 and a half teaspoons of onion powder

one fourth cup of lemon juice

one half teaspoon of garlic powder

one half or one teaspoon of cayenne pepper

1 teaspoon of lime powder

1 or 2 habanero peppers

one half teaspoon of biosalt

one half teaspoon of basil

one half teaspoon of paprika

one half teaspoon of dill

Blend until all ingredients are smooth.

Can freeze extra.

Recipe 693

CASHEW LIME ICE CREAM

Place in a vitamix the following:

The juice of a fresh coconut

1 cup of fresh coconut

½ c lime powder

3 cups of water

2 cups of walnuts

3 cups of puffed rice

2 cups of cashews

2 cups of maple syrup

1 tablespoon of almond butter

one fourth teaspoon of biosalt

Blend until smooth and pour into

one half pint jars and freeze.

Recipe 694

CASHEW WATERMELON ICE CREAM

Place in a vitamix the following:

4c watermelon

3 cups of water

2 cups of walnuts

3 cups of puffed rice

2 cups of cashews

2 cups of maple syrup

1 tablespoon of almond butter

one fourth teaspoon of biosalt

Blend until smooth and pour into

one half pint jars and freeze.

Recipe 695

CASHEW & CANTALOUPE ICE CREAM

Place in a vitamix the following:

4c Cantaloupe

3 cups of water

2 cups of walnuts

3 cups of puffed rice

2 cups of cashews

2 cups of maple syrup

1 tablespoon of almond butter

one fourth teaspoon of biosalt

Blend until smooth and pour into

one half pint jars and freeze.

Recipe 696

Cherry Tofu Cookies

FOR DOUGH: See Butter Cookie Recipe # 45

Mix the night before.

Place in refrigerator covered.

The next day place 3 cups of sucanant sugar into a vitamix. (Make into a fine powder) and pour into a large bowl.

Place 1 brick or 1 pound of tofu and 2 cups of pitted fresh cherries (remove stems)

place into a vitamix, blend until smooth.

Pour into same large bowl with sucanant sugar and add 2 cups of chopped walnuts.

Mix and set aside.

If mixture is too thin add whole wheat pastry flour, one tablespoon at a time. Roll out dough with a rolling pin and with a 3 x 3 inch round cookie cutter - cut circles into dough. Place enough mixture into cookie center and fold over, this will look like a one half moon. Press sides together and place on cookie tray lined with cookie mat.

Bake 350 degrees 20 minutes

Let cool. Store in refrigerator.

Recipe 697

STRAWBERRY TOFU COOKIES

FOR DOUGH: See Butter Cookie Recipe # 45

Mix the night before.

Place in refrigerator covered.

The next day place 3 cups of sucanant sugar into a vitamix. (Make into a fine powder) and pour into a large bowl.

Place 1 brick or 1 pound of tofu and 2 cups of strawberries (remove stems)

place into a vitamix, blend until smooth.

Pour into same large bowl with sucanant sugar and add 2 cups of chopped walnuts.

Mix and set aside.

If mixture is too thin add whole wheat pastry flour, one tablespoon at a time. Roll out dough with a rolling pin and with a 3 x 3 inch round cookie cutter - cut circles into dough. Place enough mixture into cookie center and fold over, this will look like a one half moon. Press sides together and place on cookie tray lined with cookie mat.

Bake 350 degrees 20 minutes

Let cool. Store in refrigerator.

Recipe 698

POTATO CRACKERS

Place into vitamix the following:

10 - 12 potatoes

(cleaned and remove skins)

Blend until smooth and add:

1 teaspoon of biosalt

1 teaspoon of cayenne

1 teaspoon of garlic powder

1 teaspoon of paprika

1 teaspoon of chili powder

2 tablespoons of sucanant sugar

2 tablespoons of lemon juice

2 tablespoons of lime powder or juice

Helpful hints:

The volume of batter should not fill the entire vitamix container.

So potatoes are small to medium size.

Place on oven grills overlapping 2 cookie mats per grill.

Spread thin.

Bake in oven on the lowest warm for 15 - 20 hours.

After baked store in refrigerator.

Recipe 699

SPICY HOT MUSTARD SPREAD

Place into vitamix the following:

one half cup of cashews

two thirds cup of water

2 - 4 habanero peppers (yellow or orange)

one half teaspoon of biosalt

2 teaspoons of turmeric powder

one eighth teaspoon of garlic powder

one fourth teaspoon of onion powder

8 tablespoons of lemon juice

Blend until all ingredients are smooth.

Can freeze extra.

STRAWBERRY FACE COOKIE

FILLING; Place in a vitamix the following:

1 brick or 1 pound of tofu

1 cup maple syrup

one half cup of sucanant sugar

one half cup of strawberries

1 cup of almond butter

Mix and set aside

DOUGH:

Place into a vitamix the following:

1 cup of maple syrup

one half teaspoon of vanilla

1 teaspoon of biosalt

1 teaspoon of water

one and a half cups of almond butter

Mix until smooth and add in bowl with 2 cups of whole wheat pastry flour (sifted),
    add more when needed,

Roll into balls and press into round cookie cutter 2 x 2 inches.

Cookies should look like a small pie.

Place on trays 8 per tray and into oven.

Bake 5 minutes at 375 degrees

Then place filling on top of cookies and return to oven for 5 more minutes.

Let cool. Can freeze extra.

CASHEW WALNUT CANDY

In a large bowl place the following and mix:

5 cups of cashews raw

5 cups of walnuts raw

Spay with Braggs and mix and add:

2 tablespoons of Pero

2 tablespoons of carob

Spay with Braggs, mix and add:

1 cup of maple syrup

1 cup of sucanant sugar

Mix and spray with Braggs and set aside.

Remove grill from oven. Using 2 cookie mats overlap to cover grill. Spread mixture on mats evenly. Return grill to center of oven.

Bake 12 - 24 hours on 200 degrees or until baked.

Can turn to lowest warm after 12 hours.

Recipe 702

ALMOND CAROB CANDY

Place 8 - 10 cups of raw almonds into a heavy plastic bag and with a hammer hit
each almond once to break into one half or smaller parts.

Pour into a large bowl and spray with Braggs and mix and add:

4 tablespoons of carob

Spay with Braggs, mix and add:

1 cup of maple syrup
1 cup of sucanant sugar

Mix and spray with Braggs and set aside.

Remove grill from oven. Using 2 cookie mats overlap to cover grill. Spread mixture
on mats evenly. Return grill to center of oven.

Bake 12 - 24 hours on 200 degrees or until baked.

Can turn to lowest warm after 12 hours.

PECAN CASHEW CANDY

Place in a large bowl place the following:

4 cups of pecans

4 cups of cashews raw

mix and spray with Braggs and add:

2 tablespoons of pero

2 tablespoons of carob powder

Spay with Braggs, mix and add:

1 cup of maple syrup

1 cup of sucanant sugar

Mix and spray with Braggs and set aside.

Remove grill from oven. Using 2 cookie mats overlap to cover grill. Spread mixture on mats evenly. Return grill to center of oven.

Bake 12 - 24 hours on 200 degrees or until baked.

Can turn to lowest warm after 12 hours

Recipe 704

CARAMEL CORN

Pop 8 - 10 cups of popcorn, remove seeds and one half of popped corn.

Place in a large bowl and set aside.

Place the following in a small pan and boil for 5 minutes, stirring constantly.

1 cup of almond butter

2 cups of sucanant sugar

1 cup of maple syrup

1 teaspoon of biosalt

1 teaspoon of vanilla

After 5 minutes turn heat off, let sit for

5 minutes, do not stir, after 5 minutes

stir one more time.

Pour entire mixture in a large bowl and mix - stir coating popcorn.

Then pour into a 11 x 13 inch glass dish.

Bake one hour on 250 degrees

Let cool and store in refrigerator

Recipe 705

PERO CARAMEL CORN

Pop 8 - 10 cups of popcorn, remove seeds and one half of popped corn.

Place in a large bowl and set aside.

Place the following in a small pan and boil for 5 minutes, stirring constantly.

1 - 2 tablespoons of Pero

1 cup of almond butter

2 cups of sucanant sugar

1 cup of maple syrup

1 teaspoon of biosalt

1 teaspoon of vanilla

After 5 minutes turn heat off, let sit for

5 minutes, do not stir, after 5 minutes

stir one more time.

Pour entire mixture in a large bowl and mix - stir coating popcorn.

Then pour into a 11 x 13 inch glass dish.

Bake one hour on 250 degrees

Let cool and store in refrigerator

Recipe 706

PECAN CARAMEL CORN

Pop 8 - 10 cups of popcorn, remove seeds and one half of popped corn.

Place in a large bowl and set aside.

Place the following in a small pan and boil for 5 minutes, stirring constantly.

1 cup of pecans

1 cup of almond butter

2 cups of sucanant sugar

1 cup of maple syrup

1 teaspoon of biosalt

1 teaspoon of vanilla

After 5 minutes turn heat off, let sit for

5 minutes, do not stir, after 5 minutes

stir one more time.

Pour entire mixture in a large bowl and mix - stir coating popcorn.

Then pour into a 11 x 13 inch glass dish.

Bake one hour on 250 degrees

Let cool and store in refrigerator

Recipe 707

CAROB CARAMEL CORN

Pop 8 - 10 cups of popcorn, remove seeds and one half of popped corn.

Place in a large bowl and set aside.

Place the following in a small pan and boil for 5 minutes, stirring constantly.

1 - 2 tablespoons of carob

1 cup of almond butter

2 cups of sucanant sugar

1 cup of maple syrup

1 teaspoon of biosalt

1 teaspoon of vanilla

After 5 minutes turn heat off, let sit for

5 minutes, do not stir, after 5 minutes

stir one more time.

Pour entire mixture in a large bowl and mix - stir coating popcorn.

Then pour into a 11 x 13 inch glass dish.

Bake one hour on 250 degrees

Let cool and store in refrigerator

Recipe 708

WALNUT CARAMEL CORN

Pop 8 - 10 cups of popcorn, remove seeds and one half of popped corn.

Place in a large bowl and set aside.

Place the following in a small pan and boil for 5 minutes, stirring constantly.

1 cup of chopped walnuts

1 cup of almond butter

2 cups of sucanant sugar

1 cup of maple syrup

1 teaspoon of biosalt

1 teaspoon of vanilla

After 5 minutes turn heat off, let sit for

5 minutes, do not stir, after 5 minutes

stir one more time.

Pour entire mixture in a large bowl and mix - stir coating popcorn.

Then pour into a 11 x 13 inch glass dish.

Bake one hour on 250 degrees

Let cool and store in refrigerator

Recipe 709

GUSTAVO RIOS SR. LEMON PIE COOKIES

Mix in a large bowl the following:

2 cups of sucanant sugar

one fourth cup of tofu

1 cup of almond butter

one half cup of lemon rind

Mix and add 2 cups of whole wheat pastry flour (sifted)

Mix again and place into a 9 x 9 inch cake pan, lined with parchment paper.

Press into pan with backside of a spoon.

Add one cup of chopped walnuts on top of pan; and press into dough.

Bake 275 degrees one hour

Recipe 710

DEBORAH L CERVANTES BAKED TOSTADA CASSEROLE

Place the following in a large pan and boil on low for 15 minutes.

1 can of olives

2 onions chopped

4 bell peppers chopped

4 cups of green chili peppers chopped

8 -- 12 tomatoes cut small

2 tablespoons of almond butter

1 tablespoon of chili powder

1 tablespoon of garlic powder

2 tablespoons of Braggs

1 tablespoon of Biosalt

2 teaspoons of cumin

Mix and set aside.

Place in a 9x13 inch glass dish:

6 corn tortillas "overlapping"

then add 1 cup of cooked Black beans and Pinto beans.

Spread and add one third of the above mixture and add

1 to 2 cups of any existing sauces, such as:

Pizza or Pasta sauces or a combination.

Repeat the above to add second layer,

repeat the above to add third layer.

Place a cookie mat on top of dish and place in oven.

Bake 350 degrees 30 -- 40 minutes

Serve hot.

Recipe 711

DINNER SALAD WITH TACO SHELL

For the shell see recipe # 71 (optional)

Place in shell 8 - 12 ounces of cooked pinto beans (or 2 cups)

Add enough lettuce to almost fill the top.

(tear lettuce into smaller pieces)

Place carrot flowers using a vegetable curler

(make 4)

inside flower add one thin slice of celery with one olive on top.

Add radish curl around celery using curler.

Place 2 thin slices of avocado inside each flower.

Sprinkle one long green onion cut into the top of lettuce, add 12 more olives -- cut
   into one half to decorate dish.

Add hot sauces, Braggs, or lemon juice, as much as desired.

Recipe 712

CAL EDDIE'S CINNAMON ROLLS

Place in a vitamix the following:

1 cup of soymilk

two thirds cup of sucanant sugar

two thirds cup of almond butter

2 teaspoons of biosalt

one half cup of tofu

After smooth pour into a large glass bowl, with 8 cups of whole wheat pastry flour
   (sifted) and set aside.

Yeast mixture: Place in a small bowl

one cup of finger warm water

2 packets of yeast.

2 teaspoons of sucanant sugar

Mix and add to above mixture.

Mix and knead dough.

Then place back into bowl and cover.

Place the bowl into a warm place for 1 -- 2 hours or until dough rises.

(I place in oven on the lowest warm)

Roll out dough with rolling pin and cover 3 cookie mats and in another bowl mix:

One and a half cups of sucanant sugar one and half cups of walnuts grounded one and half cups of almond butter 6 tablespoons of cinnamon Mix and spread on top of dough evenly.

Roll into a log and press sides.

Cut into one half to one inch and place in a glass dish lined with cookie mat.

Arrange each roll close together.

Bake 350 degrees for 25 - 30 minutes.

In another bowl mix:

two and a half cups of sucanant sugar
3 tablespoons of hot water
3 teaspoons of vanilla
one half cup of almond butter

Spread this mixture on top of rolls after baked.

and return to oven for 10 minutes.

Let cool and wrap and place in refrigerator 3 days before consuming.

(Place in microwave oven for 2 - 3 seconds)

Cut and serve warm.

Recipe 713

SANDY'S CINNAMON ROLLS

Place following in a vitamix:

One half cup of tofu

2 teaspoons of biosalt

1 cup of warm water

one half cup of almond butter

one half cup of sucanant sugar

mix and pour into a large bowl with 6 and a half cups of whole wheat pastry flour
sifted and set aside.

(prepare yeast) only add when above mixture is room temperature, follow yeast
instructions or place 1 tablespoon or 1 packet of yeast.

2 tablespoons of sucanant sugar

one half cup of finger warm water into a small bowl and mix. Add into the above
bowl and mix and knead.

Cover bowl and place in a warm area for 1 - 2 hours. --

(I place bowl into oven and turn to the lowest warm)

Dough will rise -- knead again.

Filling: -- In a large bowl mix the following:

4 tablespoons of cinnamon

one and a half cups of sucanant sugar

1 cup of almond butter

1 cup of chopped walnuts

Divide dough into equal halves roll out dough into a square 12x16 inches rectangle.

Can use cookie mat for size. (2 needed)

Place filling on dough and roll up and cut into 1 inch pieces.

Place in a glass baking dish 9 x 13 inches lined with cookie mat.

also place rolls close together. Let rise again in a warm place 20 -- 30 minutes.

Bake for 25 - 30 minutes at 350 degrees

Glaze : -- Mix in a bowl the following:

2 teaspoons of vanilla

2 cups of sucanant sugar

6 tablespoons of soy milk

Mix and place on top of rolls after baked, and return to oven for 5 -- 10 on broil.

Recipe 714

LEMON AND LIME DRY ROASTED CASHEWS

Place the following in a large bowl:

10 cups of raw cashew pieces

Spray -- coast with Braggs and add:

1 tablespoon of Paprika

Spray and mix with Braggs and add:

1 tablespoon of Biosalt

1 tablespoon of lime powder

1 tablespoon of lemon powder

2 tablespoons of Maple syrup

1 tablespoon of cayenne

Mix and spray with Braggs and add:

4 cups of Puffed Rice and mix and spray.

Place on oven grill lined with 2 cookie mats "overlapping".

Bake 24 hours on lowest warm or place in a fruit dryer for 6 - 8 hours.

Use 4 fruit roll trays. The above mixture will fit.

INDIAN BREAD TOSTADA

For bread: see any biscuit recipe #629 - 634

Depending on how many guests for dinner-- can double or triple recipe.

Example : I made 7 bread tostadas by using 4 times biscuit recipe. Make each the size of a tea cup dish.

Also can freeze extra after 3 days in refrigerator.

Roll out dough and place dish on top of dough and with a plastic knife cut out dough circle and place on cookie mat on trays and bake:

425 degrees for 13 - 15 minutes.

For beans: can use black or pinto. The night before:

place in a large pan 4 cups of beans and enough water to cover beans. The next day bring to boil and turn to low for 10 minutes. Change water and add one clean raw potato (after cooked throw potato away) and add:

1 onion chopped

1 bell pepper chopped

12 red or green peppers

1 cup of existing hot sauce

1 tablespoon of Braggs

1 tablespoon of chili powder

1 tablespoon of paprika

1 tablespoon of cayenne

1 tablespoon of garlic

1 teaspoon of Biosalt

1 teaspoon of maple syrup

continue to boil for 2 hours or until beans are tender.

Helpful Hints:

After 3 days can consume.

Place 6 ounces of beans on bread tostadas topped with shredded carrots for
   decoration.

Serve warm.

Recipe 716

PECAN AND WALNUT CANDY BAR

Mix in a large bowl the following:

7 cups of pecans raw

7 cups of walnuts raw

2 cups of maple syrup

2 cups of sucanant sugar

1 teaspoon of biosalt

Mix and place in a food dryer for 6 - 8 hours.

In between temperature 144 -155.

Use all 4 fruit trays and use fruit roll sheets.

After dried, let cool and place into bag and refrigerate.

Helpful Hints:

I have used Nesco American Harvest model FD61

Food Dehydrator. 1-800-288 4545

Recipe 717

OCTAVIO LEMON TART PIE COOKIES

Place the following into a *vitamix*.

1 Cup of tofu

2 tablespoons of almond butter

One and half cups of sucanant sugar

One fourth teaspoon of biosalt

1 cup of Cashews

2 -- 4 tablespoons of Lemon Powder

Mix and pour into a baked pie shell

For pie crust see Recipe # 38

Add one cup of walnuts grounded on top of pie.

Bake 10 -- 15 minutes at 400 degrees

Let cool Serve cold

Cut tart into 16 parts just like a pie.

Recipe 718

ORANGE TART PIE COOKIES

Place the following into a *vitamix*.

1 Cup of tofu

2 tablespoons of almond butter

One and half cups of sucanant sugar

One fourth teaspoon of biosalt

1 cup of Cashews

2 -- 4 tablespoons of ORANGE Powder

Mix and pour into a baked pie shell

For pie crust see Recipe # 38

Add one cup of walnuts grounded on top of pie.

Bake 10 -- 15 minutes at 400 degrees

Let cool Serve cold

Cut tart into 16 parts just like a pie.

Recipe 719

PERO TART PIE COOKIES

Place the following into a *vitamix*.

1 Cup of tofu

2 tablespoons of almond butter

One and half cups of sucanant sugar

One fourth teaspoon of biosalt

1 cup of Cashews

2 -- 4 tablespoons of pero

Mix and pour into a baked pie shell

For pie crust see Recipe # 38

Add one cup of walnuts grounded on top of pie.

Bake 10 -- 15 minutes at 400 degrees

Let cool Serve cold

Cut tart into 16 parts just like a pie.

Recipe 720

CINNAMON TART PIE COOKIES

Place the following into a *vitamix*.

1 Cup of tofu

2 tablespoons of almond butter

One and half cups of sucanant sugar

One fourth teaspoon of biosalt

1 cup of Cashews

1 - 2 tablespoons of cinnamon

Mix and pour into a baked pie shell

For pie crust see Recipe # 38

Add one cup of walnuts grounded on top of pie.

Bake 10 -- 15 minutes at 400 degrees

Let cool Serve cold

Cut tart into 16 parts just like a pie.

Recipe 721

CAROB TART PIE COOKIES

Place the following into a *vitamix*.

1 Cup of tofu

2 tablespoons of almond butter

One and half cups of sucanant sugar

One fourth teaspoon of biosalt

1 cup of Cashews

2 -- 4 tablespoons of Carob Powder

Mix and pour into a baked pie shell

For pie crust see Recipe # 38

Add one cup of walnuts grounded on top of pie.

Bake 10 -- 15 minutes at 400 degrees

Let cool Serve cold

Cut tart into 16 parts just like a pie.

Recipe 722

LIME TART PIE COOKIES

Place the following into a *vitamix*.

1 Cup of tofu

2 tablespoons of almond butter

One and half cups of sucanant sugar

One fourth teaspoon of biosalt

1 cup of Cashews

2 -- 4 tablespoons of LIME Powder

Mix and pour into a baked pie shell

For pie crust see Recipe # 38

Add one cup of walnuts grounded on top of pie

Recipe 723

VANILLA TART PIE COOKIES

Place the following into a *vitamix.*

1 Cup of tofu

2 tablespoons of almond butter

One and half cups of sucanant sugar

One fourth teaspoon of biosalt

1 cup of Cashews

`1 - 2 tablespoons of vanilla

Mix and pour into a baked pie shell

For pie crust see Recipe # 38

Add one cup of walnuts grounded on top of pie.

Bake 10 -- 15 minutes at 400 degrees

Let cool Serve cold

Recipe 724

SPICE TART PIE COOKIES

Place the following into a *vitamix*.

1 Cup of tofu

2 tablespoons of almond butter

One and half cups of sucanant sugar

One fourth teaspoon of biosalt

1 cup of Cashews

1 teaspoon of clove powder

1 teaspoon of cinnamon

1 teaspoon of ginger

Mix and pour into a baked pie shell

For pie crust see Recipe # 38

Add one cup of walnuts grounded on top of pie.

Bake 10 -- 15 minutes at 400 degrees

Let cool Serve cold

Cut tart into 16 parts just like a pie.

Recipe 725

GRAPEFRUIT TART PIE COOKIES

Place the following into a *vitamix*.

1 Cup of tofu

2 tablespoons of almond butter

One and half cups of sucanant sugar

One fourth teaspoon of biosalt

1 cup of Cashews

2 -- 4 tablespoons of grapefruit powder

Mix and pour into a baked pie shell

For pie crust see Recipe # 38

Add one cup of walnuts grounded on top of pie.

Bake 10 -- 15 minutes at 400 degrees

Let cool Serve cold

Cut tart into 16 parts just like a pie.

LICORICE TART PIE COOKIES

Place the following into a *vitamix*.

1 Cup of tofu

2 tablespoons of almond butter

One and half cups of sucanant sugar

One fourth teaspoon of biosalt

1 cup of Cashews

One fourth or one half teaspoon of liquid Anise -- depends on how strong of a licorice
taste

Mix and pour into a baked pie shell

For pie crust see Recipe # 38

Add one cup of walnuts grounded on top of pie.

Bake 10 -- 15 minutes at 400 degrees

Let cool Serve cold

Cut tart into 16 parts just like a pie.

INGREDIENTS TO AVOID

Bha-butylated bht hydroytolune

Black Strap Molasses

Caffeine

Calcium Sulfate

Carmel

Carrageen

Disodium Sulfite

Distilled water - (do not use- no minerals)

Edtacalcium disodium

Ethylenediamine

Letracetate

Gum Arabic

Cellulose chatti karaya

Gypsum

Hydroylated lecithin

Monocalcium Satisfactory Phosphate

Hydrolyzed protein

Lactic Acid

Magnesium chlorate

Maltodextrim - white sugar

Magnesium Sterate

Modified food starch

Mono+dislycerides

Mono sodium glutamate

M S G

Multol dextrin

Natural flavor

Nisarl

Non hydroxylated Lecithin

Phosforic acid

Popylgallate

Propylene Glycolalginate

Polysorbate 60, 65, 80

Red Dye 40 - Allura Red AC

Stearic Acid

Sodium Saccharin

Sodium Alginate

Sodium Benzoate

Sodium Bicarbonate

Sodium Chloride

Sodium Erythrobate

Sulfur Dioxide

Sugar black paperbicarbonate of soda

Tragacanth Xanthan

Torutein

Vinegar

Yeast flakes

RECIPES LIST

1. BAKED POTATO

2. SALADS

3. PASTA

4. PASTA SAUCE - TOMATO SAUCE

5. BROWN RICE

6. TEXAN RICE

7. BELL PEPPER RICE

8. TOSTADAS

9. POPCORN

10. HOT SAUCE

11. CINDY HUCK BEANS FOR BURRITOS

12. TODD NEUMILLER CHINESE SOUP

13. ALMOND BUTTER

14. PIZZA SAUCE

15. PIZZA DOUGH (FOR PIES)

16. WAFFLES

17. TAMALE CASSEROLE

18. MAPLE SYRUP CAKE

19. PAN - FRIED NOODLES

20. FRUIT ICING

21. CAROB BAKED ALASKA

22. VANILLA CAKE

23. CAROB GLAZE

24. MAPLE OATMEAL CAKE

25. CLOVE COOKIES

26. DONALD W. HUCK COCONUT COOKIES

27. CAROB ROMA OATMEAL COOKIES

28. DEEP - DISH PIZZA

29. COCONUT OATMEAL CAROB ROMA COOKIES

30. COCONUT OATMEAL COOKIES

31. CAROB ROMA COCONUT OATMEAL WHOLE-WHEAT PASTRY FLOUR COOKIES

32. COCONUT OATMEAL WHOLE WHEAT PASTRY FLOUR COOKIES

33. STUFFED BELL PEPPERS

34. MAPLE SYRUP COOKIES

35. CAROB COOKIES

36. CAROB BROWN CAKE

37. ANY FRUIT COOKIES (PEACH, CHERRY, APRICOT)

38. SPECIAL PIE CRUST

39. PUMPKIN PIE

40. PARVIN MALEK CAROB PIE

41. ALMOND BUTTER COOKIES 2

42. CAROB FILLING

43. EVELYN ANN MENZIE OLD-FASHIONED GLAZE

44. PINEAPPLE PIE

45. BUTTER COOKIES

46. SUCANANT COOKIES

47. INEZ A. MENZIE COCONUT COOKIES

48. TURNOVERS

49. GOLDEN MACAROONS

50. ORIENTAL CRUNCH

51. PINEAPPLE CANDY

52. CAROB DOUGHNUTS

53. LEMON DOUGHNUTS

54. GRAIN PIZZA

55. CORNMEAL PIZZA

56. CAROB BROWNIES

57. ROBERT E MENZIE WALNUT PIE

58. APRICOT COCONUT WALNUT SQUARES

59. PISTACHIO SCONES

60. EGG ROLLS

61. ROASTED SALTED NUTS

62. FUDGE CUP COOKIE

63. FUDGE SAUCE

64. PINEAPPLE COOKIES

65. TAMALE BEAN PIE

66. NUT PIE

67. DATE WALNUT COOKIES

68. CARAMELIZED GINGER HAZELNUT TART

69. PAPAYA COOKIES

70. CAJUN MIXED NUTS

71. TACO SALAD SHELLS

72. FOR CAKE-WEDDING STYLE CAKE

73. SPANISH MILLET CASSEROLE

74. ENCHILADAS

75. CAROB PIE

76. NUT BUTTER BALLS

77. SHARAREH SHABAFROOZ GARLIC BREAD SPREAD/BUTTER

78. GLAZED CARROT CAKE

79. WAFFLES WITH CASHEWS AND OATMEAL

80. LEMON PINEAPPLE PIE

81. CORN BREAD

82. MATTHEW F. MOONEY ROAST FOR ANY HOLIDAY

83. SPICE DOUGHNUTS

84. SPANISH RICE

85. PINEAPPLE SANDWICH COOKIE

86. CAROB CUP COOKIE

87. ANY FRUIT CUP COOKIE

88. SETAREH TAIS CAKE

89. CAROB DATE PISTACHIO PASTRY

90. FRUIT CAKE COOKIE

91. BAKED MILLET

92. BISCOTTI

93. MULTIGRAIN CRACKERS

94. POT PIE

95. BASIC COOKIE WITH FROSTING

96. TACO SHELLS

97. ANY FRUIT PASTRY

98. PINEAPPLE FROSTING

99. PINEAPPLE UPSIDE DOWN CAKE

100. HOT BEANS FOR BURRITOS

101. APRICOT PIE

102. APPLE PIE

103. PLUM PIE

104. PIZZA SAUCE NO. 3

105. PIZZA SAUCE NO. 1

106. COFFEE MUFFINS

107. GLORIA DUGGINS PECAN CANDY

108. PETER P. PANAGOPOULOS ALMOND FUDGE

109. PETE/ROSA CERRILLO CINNAMON WALNUT CANDY

110. SUGARED NUTS

111. PAPAYA CANDY

112. CAROB CAKE

113. THELMA MAIN HAZELNUT FUDGE

114. WHEAT CORNMEAL PIZZA

115. MARGARET/HARVEY BINDER PECAN FUDGE

116. MICHAEL F. MOONEY PECAN ROMA CAROB CANDY

117. BELLE HUCK WALNUT FUDGE

118. SAUCE FOR INSIDE CINNAMON ROLLS

119. NECTARINE PIE

120. COOKIES/CAROB PLAIN OR ROMA

121. CAROB BARS

122. SPICE BUTTER COOKIES

123. OAT CRACKERS

124. CINNAMON SUGAR DOUGHNUT TOPPING

125. JELLY DOUGHNUT FILLING

126. STRUDEL DOUGH

127. DATE CUP COOKIE

128. ITALIAN SAUCE

129 LASAGNA

130. BOB PANAGOPOULOS PIZZA SAUCE NO. 2

131. CUBAN BLACK BEANS IN RICE

132. BLACK BEANS

133. LIGHT FUDGE

134. DARK FUDGE

135. PIGEON BEANS

136. XENIA PANAGOPOULOS PIGEON RICE

137. ALEXANDRA PANAGOPOULOS SWEET AND SOUR SAUCE NO. 1

138. INEZ SPEIDELL SWEET AND SOUR SAUCE NO. 2

139. VERY VERY HOT SAUCE

140. LENTILS

141. SHRIMP SAUCE

142. ALMOND CAROB CANDY

143. CAROB ROMA CANDY

144. WALNUT CINNAMON CLUSTERS

145. TAMARA NEUMILLER SPANISH PASTA

146. CHINESE RICE

147. CHILI BEANS

148. TAMALES

149. VEGETABLE SOUP

150. CAROB ROMA COOKIES

151. RAY AND LINDA PANAGOPOULOS SUNFLOWER COCONUT WAFFLES

152. WAFFLES OATMEAL AND ALMONDS

153. RHI CAROB AND ROMA OATMEAL WWP NUTLESS COOKIE

154. HOT SAUCE

155. RED BEANS FOR TOP OF RICE

156. CORNMEAL WAFFLES

157. TAGLIATELLE SAUCE

158. ALMOND BUTTER COOKIES

159. MAPLE SYRUP FROSTING

160. ORANGE GLAZE

161. RYE PANCAKES

162. PANCAKES

163. BLUEBERRY TOPPING

164. ROMA ICE CREAM

165. LEMON ICE CREAM

166. ORANGE DATE SYRUP

167. CAROB FUDGE SAUCE

168. COCONUT LIME FROSTING

169. CREAMY FROSTING

170. WHIPPED CREAM

171 COCONUT CREAM TOPPING NO. 1

172 COCONUT CREAM TOPPING NO. 2

173 MOHAMAD-TAGHI MALEK CAROB MOUSSE

174 CATSUP NO. 1

175 CAROB ROMA ALMOND CANDY

176 ANGEL MACAROONS

177 NUT MILK

178 ROMA PIE

179 MUSTARD SPREAD

180 CAROB ROMA FROSTING

181 BASIC FROSTING

182 CAROB ROMA COCONUT COOKIES

183 CAROB ICE CREAM

184 CAROB CARAMEL BARS

185 CAROB SYRUP

186 CAROB COCONUT FROSTING

187 SPECIAL SEASONING FOR ANYTHING

188 ITALIAN SALAD DRESSING

189 PINEAPPLE ICE CREAM

190 ORANGE ICE CREAM

191 CATSUP EXTRA

192 CHERRY ICE CREAM

193 THESE COLORS TO BE USED WITH WHIPPED CREAM (SEE RECIPE NO.170) REAL COLORS FOR CAKES AND COOKIES

194 CAROB PUDDING OR PIE FILLING

195 ENGLISH TOFFEE COOKIE

196 CAROB CAKE FROSTING

197 COCONUT CAKE

198 PUMPKIN COOKIES

199 MARSELLAS PANAGOPOULOS BRAZIL NUT ICE CREAM

200 TAHEREH MALEK PUMPKIN ICE CREAM

201 BAKED BROWN RICE

202 GINGER CANDY

203 SANDY MOONEY COFFEE CAKE

204 PAPAYA WALNUT COOKIES

205 LEMON CARROT COOKIES

206 CAROB SANDWICH COOKIES

207 DAISY FROSTING

208 BLACK-EYED PEAS

209 ALMOND BUTTER FROSTING

210 CRUNCH TOPPING FOR ANY BAKED PIE

211 CHERI GILBERT COOKED CAROB GLAZE

212 SUCANANT SUGAR GLAZE

213 ROMA CREAM FROSTING

214 LEMON FILLING

215 BAR-B-QUE SAUCE

216 TOFU FROSTING

217 SWEET SUGAR ICING

218 BLACK EYED IN RICE

219 SOY MILK CORNBREAD

220 OATMEAL ALMOND COOKIE

221 SPICED CUPCAKES

222 DATE OATMEAL COOKIE

223 ORANGE COCONUT COOKIE

224 DATE COOKIE BAR

225 APRICOT COOKIE BAR

226 GINGER PANCAKES

227 LEMON PASTRY

228 LEMON SUGAR COOKIES

229 DATE BROWNIES

230 ORIGINAL SALT WATER TAFFY

231 AURA VICTORIA HUCK PEPPERMINT SALT WATER TAFFY

232 LEMON SALT WATER TAFFY

233 VANILLA SALT WATER TAFFY

234 ORANGE SALT WATER TAFFY

235 JACK PANAGOPOULOS ROMA SALT WATER TAFFY

236 ADRIANA CERRILLO PECAN SALT WATER TAFFY

237 ELMER LYLE MENZIE ALMOND SALT WATER TAFFY

238 ASHLEY SPEIDELL WALNUT SALT WATER TAFFY

239 ROSS H. MENZIE CAROB SALT WATER TAFFY

240 COCONUT SALT WATER TAFFY

241 CINNAMON SALT WATER TAFFY

242 GINGER SALT WATER TAFFY

243 GENE KOENIG ENGLISH TOFFEE CANDY

244 LUCILLE GILBERT LEMON CHEESECAKE

245 ORANGE CHEESECAKE

246 ASHER MICHAEL NEUMILLER CAROB CHEESECAKE

247 ALLIE NICOLE BLUMA NEUMILLER CAROB CAKE

248 DR. EDE VANILLA SUGAR CAKE

249 WALNUT SQUARE COOKIES

250 TARA SHABAFROOZ PECAN SQUARE COOKIES

251 ALMOND SQUARE COOKIES

252 MARGARET ANN MENZIE PECAN ROPE COOKIES

253 MASSOOD SHABAFROOZ WALNUT ROPE COOKIES

254 ALMOND ROPE COOKIES

255 RHI COCONUT OATMEAL CAROB AND ROMA COOKIES

256 RHI COCONUT OATMEAL COOKIES

257 RHI COCONUT OATMEAL WHOLE WHEAT PASTRY FLOUR COOKIES

258 RHI CAROB COCONUT COOKIES

259 RHI COCONUT COOKIES

260 RHI CAROB AND ROMA OATMEAL COOKIES

261 RHI VANILLA DONUTS OR CAKE

262 RHI CAROB BROWN CAKE

263 RHI GOLDEN MACAROONS

291 POCKET APRICOT PASTRY

292 POCKET CHERRY PASTRY

293 POCKET PEACH PASTRY

294 POCKET PINEAPPLE - LEMON PASTRY

295 POCKET PUMPKIN PASTRY

296 POCKET APPLE PASTRY

297 POCKET EGG ROLLS

298 POCKET BEAN BURRITO

299 APRICOT CREAM PIE

300 VERA WALDSCHMIDT CHERRY CREAM PIE

301 PEACH CREAM PIE

302 APPLE CREAM PIE

303 TAHEREH TAHERIAN HABANERO HOT SAUCE

304 SHAHNAZ SHAINEE HOT AND SPICY PINTO BEANS

305 PAYAM MALEK ZADEH CAROB WHEAT COOKIES

306 RAISIN ICE CREAM

307 TOMATO CASSEROLE

308 RAISIN FACE COOKIE

309 DATE FACE COOKIE

310 PINEAPPLE COCONUT SQUARES

311 ORANGE PINEAPPLE ICE CREAM

312 LEMON PINEAPPLE ICE CREAM

313 ROMA FACE COOKIE

314 CAROB FACE COOKIE

315 PUMPKIN FACE COOKIE

316 PINEAPPLE FACE COOKIE

317 APPLE FACE COOKIE

318 PEACH FACE COOKIE

319 APRICOT FACE COOKIE

320 PLUM FACE COOKIE

321 CHERRY FACE COOKIE

322 WALNUT DOME COOKIES

323 ALMOND DOME COOKIES

324 PECAN DOME COOKIES

325 CAROB DOME COOKIES

326 ROMA DOME COOKIES

327 COFFEE CUP COOKIE

328 RAISIN CUP COOKIE

329 WALNUT CUP COOKIE

330 POCKET PASTA NO. 4

331 POCKET PASTA NO. 2

332 POCKET PASTA NO. 3

333 POCKET PASTA NO. 1

334 BRAZIL NUT CARAMEL CANDY

335 HABANERO BAKED RICE

336 MACADAMIA CARAMEL CANDY

337 CINNAMON CARAMEL CANDY

338 WALNUT CARAMEL CANDY

339 COCONUT CARAMEL CANDY

340 PECAN CARAMEL CANDY

341 PISTACHIO CARAMEL CANDY

342 HAZELNUT CARAMEL CANDY

343 CASHEW CARAMEL CANDY

344 ROASTED ALMOND CARAMEL CANDY

345 LEMON CARAMEL CANDY

346 ORANGE CARAMEL CANDY

347 CAROB CARAMEL CANDY

348 ROMA CARMEL CANDY

349 PEPPERMINT CARAMEL CANDY

350 GINGER CARAMEL CANDY

351 HERBS & GARLIC BAKED RICE

352 WALNUT & ALMOND FROSTING

353 PINEAPPLE & LEMON GLAZE

354 ROMA TOFU COOKIES

355 CAROB TOFU COOKIES

356 CINNAMON TOFU COOKIES

357 RAISIN TOFU COOKIES

358 APRICOT TOFU COOKIES

359 DATE TOFU COOKIES

360 CRANBERRY TOFU COOKIES

361 SPICE TOFU COOKIES

362 PAPAYA TOFU COOKIES

363 COCONUT TOFU COOKIES

364 LEMON TOFU COOKIES

365 ORANGE TOFU COOKIES

366 PINEAPPLE TOFU COOKIES

367 BLACK BEAN SOUP

368 LEMON COCONUT COOKIES

369 CHERRY SUGAR COOKIES

370 ORANGE SUGAR COOKIES

371 RAISIN SUGAR COOKIES

372 ROMA SUGAR COOKIES

373 APPLE SUGAR COOKIES

374 CAROB SUGAR COOKIES

375 PEPPERMINT SUGAR COOKIES

376 BLUEBERRY SUGAR COOKIE

377 DATE SUGAR COOKIE

378 PINEAPPLE SUGAR COOKIE

379 PLUM SUGAR COOKIE

380 PEACH SUGAR COOKIE

381 APRICOT SUGAR COOKIE

382 NECTARINE SUGAR COOKIE

383 CRANBERRY SUGAR COOKIE

384 PUMPKIN SUGAR COOKIE

385 COCONUT CAROB CARAMEL CANDY

386 COCONUT LEMON CARAMEL CANDY

387 COCONUT CINNAMON CARAMEL CANDY

388 COCONUT ORANGE CARAMEL CANDY

389 COCONUT PEPPERMINT CARAMEL CANDY

390 COCONUT ROMA CARMEL CANDY

391 COCONUT GINGER CARAMEL CANDY

392 DATE OATMEAL COOKIE

393 RAISIN OATMEAL COOKIE

394 WALNUT DATE COOKIE

395 WALNUT LEMON COOKIE

396 WALNUT RAISIN COOKIE

397 WALNUT ORANGE COOKIE

398 WALNUT CHERRY COOKIE

399 COCONUT DATE COOKIE

400 COCONUT CHERRY COOKIE

401 COCONUT RAISIN COOKIE

402 ONION DRIED ROASTED NUTS

403 GARLIC DRIED ROASTED NUTS

404 HABANERO DRIED ROASTED NUTS

405 CAYENNE DRIED ROASTED NUTS

406 BLACK BEAN RICE

407 SALTED-HABANERO DRIED ROASTED NUT MIX

408 MAPLE SYRUP DRIED ROASTED NUTS

409 CAROB MACAROONS

410 LEMON MACAROONS

411 ROMA MACAROONS

412 ORANGE MACAROONS

413 PEPPERMINT FROSTING

414 PINEAPPLE-LEMON BAKED ALASKA

415 LEMON BAKED ALASKA

416 ORANGE BAKED ALASKA

417 PEPPERMINT BAKED ALASKA

418 VANILLA BAKED ALASKA

419 RED HOT FIRE SAUCE

420 APRICOT ICE CREAM

421 TWICE COOKED HERB POTATO

422 PEPPERMINT MACARONS

423 PEACH ICE CREAM

424 TWICE COOKED SPICY POTATO

425 PLUM MACAROONS

426	SPICY GARLIC SPREAD
427	ITALIAN SPREAD
428	WALNUT WAFFLES
429	POPPY SEED WAFFLES
430	PUMPKIN SEED WAFFLES
431	CAROB SUCANAT SUGAR COOKIE
432	ROMA SUCANAT SUGAR COOKIE
433	PEPPERMINT SUCANAT SUGAR COOKIE
434	CINNAMON SUCANAT SUGAR COOKIE
435	GINGER SUCANAT SUGAR COOKIE
436	CAROB SUGARED NUTS
437	ROMA SUGARED NUTS
438	PECAN PIE
439	BLUEBERRY CREAM PIE
440	GRAPE PIE
441	LEMON FROSTING
442	ORANGE CAKE FROSTING
443	VANILLA CAKE FROSTING
444	PEACH MAPLE CAKE
445	PLUM MAPLE CAKE
446	APRICOT MAPLE CAKE
447	PINEAPPLE MAPLE CAKE
448	APPLE MAPLE CAKE
449	CHERRY MAPLE CAKE
450	NECTARINE MAPLE CAKE
451	LEMON MAPLE CAKE
452	ORANGE MAPLE CAKE

453 BLUEBERRY MAPLE CAKE

454 PEAR MAPLE CAKE

455 BLUEBERRY BAKED ALASKA

456 BARBEQUE HOT SAUCE

457 PISTACHIO WAFFLES

458 PEACH BAKED ALASKA

459 APRICOT BAKED ALASKA

460 APPLE BAKED ALASKA

461 PLUM BAKED ALASKA

462 NECTARINE BAKED ALASKA

463 GRAPE BAKED ALASKA

464 CHEESE SAUCE FOR BAKED POTATO

465 APPLE ICE CREAM

466 PLUM ICE CREAM

467 GRAPE ICE CREAM

468 PEAR ICE CREAM

469 RHI MAPLE SYRUP COOKIES

470 MAPLE SYRUP BROWNIES

471 CAROB NUGGET CANDY

472 ROMA NUGGET CANDY

473 PEPPERMINT NUGGET CANDY

474 CINNAMON NUGGET CANDY

475 LEMON NUGGET CANDY

476 VANILLA NUGGET

477 APRICOT NUGGET CANDY

478 ITALIAN DRY ROASTED NUT MIX

479 GARLIC DRY ROASTED PUFF CORN MIX

480 ONION DRY ROASTED PUFF CORN MIX

481 HABANERO DRY ROASTED PUFF CORN MIX

482 CAYENNE DRY ROASTED PUFF CORN MIX

483 ITALIAN DRY ROASTED PUFF CORN MIX

484 SALTED DRY ROASTED PUFF CORN MIX

485 CAJUN DRY ROASTED PUFF CORN MIX

486 SALTED HABANERO DRY ROASTED PUFF C CORN MIX

487 PLUM TOFU COOKIES

488 PEACH TOFU COOKIES

489 NECTARINE TOFU COOKIES

490 SPICY AVOCADO DIP

491 ALL-PURPOSE GRAVY

492 POTATO AND CABBAGE STEW

493 CAROB PIE CRUST

494 ROMA PIE CRUST

495 COFFEE BAKED PIE

496 CRANBERRY SAUCE

497 GREEN BEANS CASSEROLE

498 QUICK OATMEAL

499 BAKED YAMS

500 SAUTÉ CORN

501 CINNAMON AND GINGER COOKIES

502 ORANGE NUGGET CANDY

503 POTATO AND CELERY SOUP

504 AVOCADO DIP

505 CARROT SOUP

506 PEACH UPSIDE DOWN CREAM CAKE

507 APRICOT UPSIDE DOWN CREAM CAKE

508 NECTARINE UPSIDE DOWN CREAM CAKE

509 CHERRY UPSIDE DOWN CREAM CAKE

510 GRAPE UPSIDE DOWN CREAM CAKE

511 APPLE UPSIDE DOWN CREAM CAKE

512 CINNAMON UPSIDE DOWN CREAM CAKE

513 CAROB UPSIDE DOWN CREAM CAKE

514 PLUM UPSIDE DOWN CREAM CAKE

515 ROMA UPSIDE DOWN CREAM CAKE

516 PINEAPPLE UPSIDE DOWN CREAM CAKE

517 PEPPERMINT UPSIDE DOWN CREAM CAKE

518 ORANGE UPSIDE DOWN CREAM CAKE

519 LEMON UPSIDE DOWN CREAM CAKE

520 GINGER UPSIDE DOWN CREAM CAKE

521 JAMAICAN RICE

522 LEMON AND OLIVE BASMATI RICE MIX

523 CARROT AND OLIVE BASMATI RICE MIX

524 GARLIC AND ONION SAUTÉED CORN

525 GREEN JALAPENO RICE MIX

526 ROASTED PISTACHIO CANDY

527 PISTACHIO FUDGE

528 SPICY CORN BREAD

529 RED HOT ROAST

530 CINNAMON WALNUT COOKIES

531 ORANGE BALL COOKIES

532 LEMON BALL COOKIES

533 ORANGE PASTRY

534 CINNAMON MACARONS

535 CINNAMON AND OATMEAL COOKIES

536 RED POTATO CASSEROLE

537 CINNAMON ICE CREAM

538 DATE WALNUT TART

539 WALNUT GINGER COOKIES

540 WALNUT ROMA COOKIES

541 WALNUT CAROB COOKIES

542 SPICE WALNUT COOKIES

543 LEMON AND HERB DRY ROASTED NUT MIX

544 LEMON AND DILL DRY ROASTED NUT MIX

545 LEMON AND SALTED DRY ROASTED NUT MIX

546 SWEET AND SOUR DRY ROASTED NUT MIX

547 LEMON AND CAYENNE DRY ROASTED NUT MIX

548 LEMON AND CAJUN DRY ROASTED NUT MIX

549 LEMON AND HABANERO DRY ROASTED NUT MIX

550 LEMON AND ONION DRY ROASTED NUT MIX

551 LEMON AND GARLIC DRY ROASTED NUT MIX

552 NECTARINE ICE CREAM

553 SPICE ICE CREAM

554 THIN CORN BREAD

555 NECTARINE CREAM PIE

556 CINNAMON PIE

557 CINNAMON CHEESECAKE

558 CINNAMON DATE PASTRY

559 CARAMELIZED CINNAMON TART

560 CINNAMON CANDY

561 LICORICE ICE CREAM

562 LICORICE FROSTING

563 LICORICE BAKED ALASKA

564 LICORICE CHEESE CAKE

565 LICORICE TOFFEE COOKIES

566 LICORICE FUDGE

567 LICORICE SALT WATER TOFFEE

568 LICORICE COCONUT CARAMELS

569 LICORICE CANDY

570 LICORICE COCONUT COOKIES

571 LICORICE MACARONS

572 HABANERO RICE

573 MARTIN MASSOOD LICORICE SANDWICH COOKIES

574 CINNAMON SANDWICH COOKIES

575 CORN ON THE COB

576 AVA DANIELLE NEUMILLER ORANGE CREAM PIE

577 CINNAMON WALNUT FUDGE

578 WALNUT CRUST FOR ANY PIE

579 GREEN PEAS AND RICE

580 LEMON CREAM PIE

581 COCONUT CREAM PIE

582 PUMPKIN AND APPLE COOKIES

583 SUCANANT FACE COOKIES

584 HAZELNUT FACE COOKIES

585 HAZELNUT CAROB COOKIES

586 PISTACHIO FACE COOKIES

587 PILAF RICE MIX

588 PERO SUCANANT COOKIES

589 HAZELNUT SPICE COOKIES

590 CINNAMON WALNUT FACE COOKIES

591 CAROB-COCONUT FACE COOKIES

592 LEMON WALNUT COOKIES

593 ORANGE WALNUT COOKIES

594 ANISE WALNUT COOKIES

595 PEPPERMINT WALNUT COOKIES

596 CAROB COCONUT PIE COOKIES

597 PERO AND HAZELNUT PIE COOKIES

598 CARAMELIZED CINNAMON PISTACHIO TART

599 VITAMIX LICORICE MACARONS

600 VITAMIX CINNAMON MACARONS

601 VITAMIX PEPPERMINT MACARONS

602 WIN TINSON STRAWBERRY CREAM PIE

603 STRAWBERRY ICE CREAM

604 STRAWBERRY CHEESE CAKE

605 BLUEBERRY CHEESE CAKE

606 STRAWBERRY BAKED ALASKA

607 STRAWBERRY MAPLE CAKE

608 STRAWBERRY UPSIDE DOWN CREAM CAKE

609 FIRE DRY ROASTED NUT MIX

610 CITRUS AND HERB RICE

611 BARBEQUE SEASONED RICE

612 MEXICAN SEASONED RICE

613 JAMAICAN SEASONED RICE

614 ITALIAN SEASONED RICE

615 TACO SEASONED RICE

616 THAI SEASONED RICE

617 PIZZA SEASONED RICE

618 CAJUN SEASONED RICE

619 ORIENTAL SEASONED RICE

620 CAROB CASHEW CREAM PIE

621 PERO CASHEW CREAM PIE

622 CINNAMON CASHEW CREAM PIE

623 LEMON CASHEW CREAM PIE

624 ORANGE CASHEW CREAM PIE

625 SPICE CASHEW CREAM PIE

626 LICORICE AND CASHEW CREAM PIE

627 GREEN HOT SAUCE

628 GREEN SALSA

629 SESAME SEED BISCUITS

630 ITALIAN BISCUITS

631 GARLIC BISCUITS

632 HOT BISCUITS

633 SOYMILK BISCUITS

634 POPPY SEED BISCUITS

635 GUSTAVO RIOS SR LEMON PIE COOKIES

636 HORTENCIA RIOS SPICE PIE COOKIES

637 ORANGE PIE COOKIES

638 DATE PIE COOKIES

639 CASHEW AND CAROB ICE CREAM

640 CASHEW-CAROB-ROMA ICE CREAM

641 CASHEW-PUMPKIN-ICE CREAM

642 CASHEW ORANGE ICE CREAM

643 CASHEW-PINEAPPLE-ICE CREAM

644 CASHEW RAISIN ICE CREAM

645 CASHEW APRICOT ICE CREAM

646 CASHEW LICORICE ICE CREAM

647 CASHEW SPICE ICE CREAM

648 CASHEW ROMA ICE CREAM

649 CASHEW LEMON ICE CREAM

650 CASHEW CINNAMON ICE CREAM

651 CASHEW PEPPERMINT ICE CREAM

652 CASHEW ROMA PEPPERMINT ICE CREAM

653 CASHEW BLACKBERRY ICE CREAM

654 CASHEW CHERRY ICE CREAM

655 CASHEW NECTARINE ICE CREAM

656 CASHEW STRAWBERRY ICE CREAM

657 CASHEW PEACH ICE CREAM

658 CASHEW ORANGE PINEAPPLE ICE CREAM

659 CASHEW LEMON PINEAPPLE ICE CREAM

660 LEMON SUCANANT SUGAR COOKIES

661 ORANGE SUCANANT SUGAR COOKIES

662 COCONUT CASHEW CREAM PIE

663 PLUM FRUIT ROLL

664 CHERRY FRUIT ROLL

665 LICORICE PLUM FRUIT ROLL

666 DATE AND PLUM ICE CREAM

667 GRAPEFRUIT ICE CREAM

668 PEACH FRUIT ROLL

669   APRICOT FRUIT ROLL

670   STRAWBERRY FRUIT ROLL

671   PEAR FRUIT ROLL

672   NECTARINE FRUIT ROLL

673   BLACKBERRY FRUIT ROLL

674   PINEAPPLE FRUIT ROLL

675   APPLE FRUIT ROLL

676   ORANGE PLUM FRUIT ROLL

677   LEMON PLUM FRUIT ROLL

678   GRAPEFRUIT PLUM FRUIT ROLL

679   PEPPERMINT PLUM FRUIT ROLL

680   MARK D DAWSON ASIAN HOT SAUCE

681   GREEN ASIAN HOT SAUCE

682   VANILLA FRUIT ROLL

683   CASHEW COCONUT ICE CREAM

684   COCONUT ICE CREAM

685   CANTALOUPE FRUIT ROLL

686   MANGO FRUIT ROLL

687   PAPAYA FRUIT ROLL

688   GREEN HABANERO & RED PEPPER HOT SAUCE

689   HABANERO & RED PEPPER HOT SAUCE

690   CHERRY AND HABANERO RICE

691   LEMON-ORANGE-LIME GRAPEFRUIT POWDER

692   SPICY CATSUP

693   CASHEW LIME ICE CREAM

694   GABRIEL CERRILLO WATERMELON ICE CREAM

695   CASHEW CANTALOUPE ICE CREAM

696   CHERRY TOFU COOKIES

697   STRAWBERRY TOFU COOKIES

698   POTATO CRACKERS

699   SPICY HOT MUSTARD SPREAD

700   STRAWBERRY FACE COOKIES

701   CASHEW WALNUT CANDY

702   ALMOND CAROB CANDY

703   PECAN CASHEW CANDY

704   CARAMEL CORN

705   PERO CARAMEL CORN

706   PECAN CARAMEL CORN

707   CAROB CARAMEL CORN

708   WALNUT CARAMEL CORN

709   GUSTAVO RIOS SR. LEMON PIE COOKIES

710   DEBORAH CERVANTES BAKED TOSTADA CASSEROLE

711   DINNER SALAD WITH TACO SHELLS

712   CAL EDDIE'S CINNAMON ROLLS

713   SANDRA'S CINNAMON ROLLS

714   LEMON AND LIME DRY ROASTED CASHEWS

715   INDIAN BREAD TOSTADA

716   PECAN AND WALNUT CANDY BAR

717   OCTAVIO LEMON TART PIE COOKIES

718   ORANGE TART PIE COOKIES

719   PERO TART PIE COOKIES

720   CINNAMON TART PIE COOKIES

721   CAROB TART PIE COOKIES

722   LIME TART PIE COOKIES

CONCLUSION

You and only you can take control for the responsibility of your health which is so important.

You owe it to yourself and your loved ones to be healthy and disease free.

All it takes is commitment on your part to be healthy and eat properly. By incorporating the information that I have provided for you in this book, you will probably never, or rarely, ever need the service of a medical or natural pathic doctor. I am a living testimonial to the fact that real food – food that is full of nutrition, that will not harm your body – and having a clean colon will provide good health. It has helped me to become healthy and it will most certainly help everyone to gain and / or retain good health. I have gone from a very unhealthy person to someone who has virtually no health problems. I no longer have to live with diabetes, kidney stones, bone problems, or being overweight. The fifty-five pounds that I have lost has never come back, and I have no problems in maintaining proper weight. I am certain that all of my poor health problems would have only been maintained or gotten worse if I were under a doctor's care and had not taken responsibility for my own health. I would have had major or minor operations, taken many drugs and suffered from the great number of side effects and have had a poor quality of life. But instead I am having a life free of pain, suffering, and limitations.

I am so excited about my discoveries of good health and enjoying sharing my research with others that I have now written eight books and developed over two thousand delicious recipes that have won over one-hundred cooking contests. I enjoy sharing my on going positive experiences of good health in the hopes that I can help others achieve the life quality that took me thousands of hours of research to achieve. It is exciting and amazing on how easy it is to have a healthy body.

This amounts to thousands of hours of research, experiments. and interviews. These procedures could not have taken place as an unhealthy person, based on the time and expense alone.

I have so many positive experiences that have happened and continue to enter my life after becoming healthy, it is totally amazing and exciting.

Just being healthy is for everyone and not just the few. Being healthy comes with the realization that most people including family and friends are living a life of pain and suffering. It is very predictable where they are headed, and is sad to see what they do not realize. The worst part of this situation is that being healthy is not an easy task. Everything will affect your body, mind, finances, savings, having extra time, consuming delicious foods, and more. It is time for you to give up the negative lifestyle and trade it for a positive lifestyle full of benefits.

REFERENCES

Ede Koenig M.D., Founder and Director of the Radiant Health Institute

Milton G. Crane M.D.

Kirk Donsabach M.D.